the
sex
inspectors
masterclass

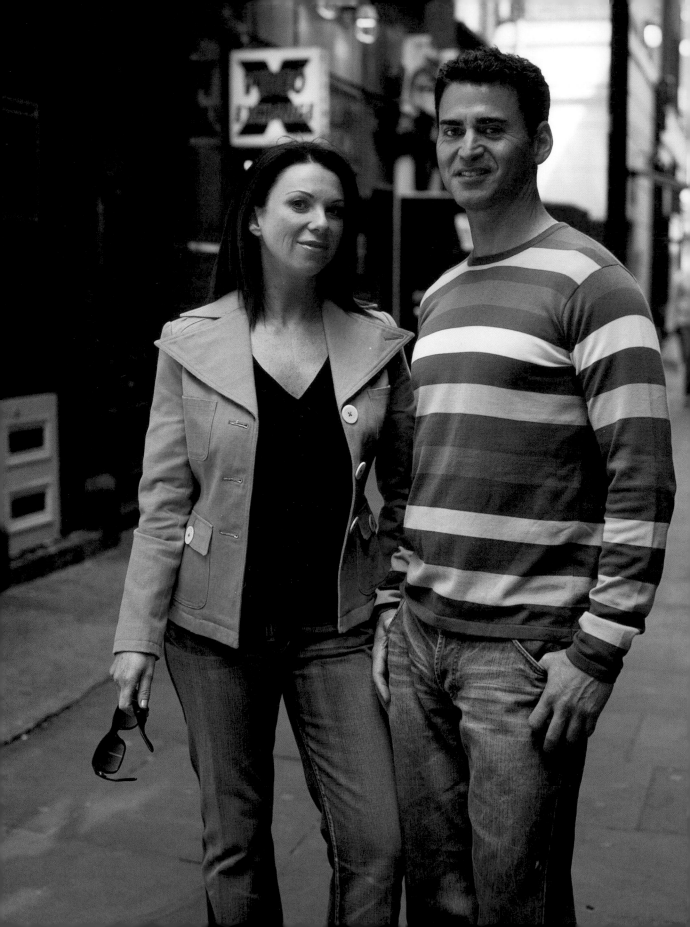

the
sex
inspectors
masterclass

Tracey Cox & Michael Alvear

illustrations by natasha law

photography by chris tubbs; still life photography by benoit audureau

MICHAEL JOSEPH
an imprint of penguin books

To all the couples who invited us into their homes. You have helped many others

MICHAEL JOSEPH

Published by the Penguin Group
Penguin Books Ltd, 80 Strand, London WC2R 0RL, England
Penguin Group (USA) Inc., 375 Hudson Street, New York, New York 10014, USA
Penguin Group (Canada), 90 Eglinton Avenue East, Suite 700, Toronto, Ontario, Canada M4P 3YZ
(a division of Pearson Penguin Canada Inc.)
Penguin Ireland, 25 St Stephen's Green, Dublin 2, Ireland (a division of Penguin Books Ltd)
Penguin Group (Australia), 250 Camberwell Road,
Camberwell, Victoria 3124, Australia (a division of Pearson Australia Group Pty Ltd)
Penguin Books India Pvt Ltd, 11 Community Centre,
Panchsheel Park, New Delhi – 110 017, India
Penguin Group (NZ), cnr Airborne and Rosedale Roads, Albany,
Auckland 1310, New Zealand (a division of Pearson New Zealand Ltd)
Penguin Books (South Africa) (Pty) Ltd, 24 Sturdee Avenue,
Rosebank 2196, Johannesburg, South Africa

Penguin Books Ltd, Registered Offices: 80 Strand, London WC2R 0RL, England

www.penguin.com

First published 2005
1

Text copyright © Fremantle Media Ltd, 2005

The moral right of the authors has been asserted

Always practise safe and responsible sex, and consult a doctor if you have any condition
that precludes strenuous sexual activity. The author and publisher do not accept any
responsibility for any ailment or injury caused by the information contained in this book.

Set in Univers
Designed and typeset by NIKKI DUPIN
Printed in Great Britain by Butler and Tanner, Frome

A CIP catalogue record for this book is available from the British Library

ISBN 0–718–14851–7

contents

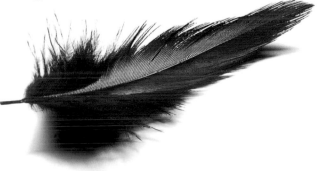

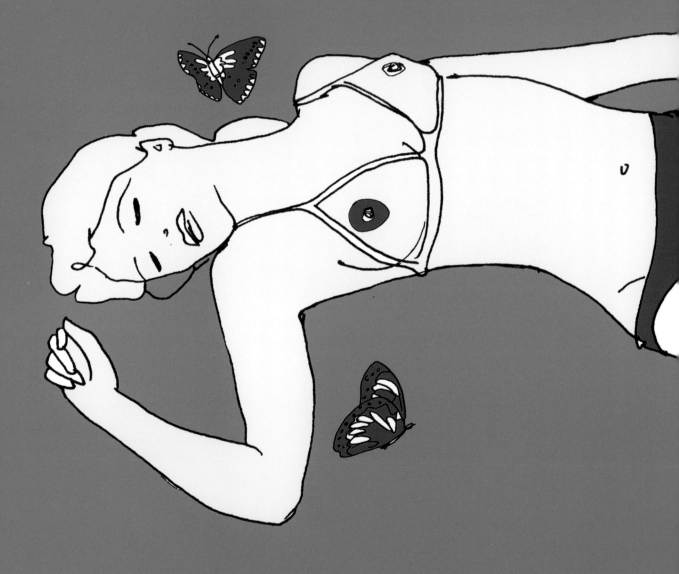

introduction

IT WAS THE FIRST SHOOT OF THE SEX INSPECTORS, the bit where we watch recorded footage of the couples having sex. I tried to be cool, unshockable, the consummate professional. I really did. But I still ended up watching that first tape through my fingers, mouth open, jaw on the floor, squirming and half-hiding behind my co-presenter Michael Alvear. Apparently, this wasn't quite what our executive producer, Steph Harris, was looking for. 'Let's stop a minute,' she said, biting her lip. 'Umm, Trace, is it possible for you to look a little less – how do I put this? – prudish while you're watching the couples? I mean, you are a sexpert. And it is a show about sex. So you have to expect, well, to see some occasionally.'

She had a point. I knew the deal when I said yes to the show and I totally agree with the logic behind putting the cameras in to record each couple's love life. Most of us are too emotionally involved to report objectively about our sex lives. We can be shrewd and perceptive, maybe, but it's almost impossible not to be subjective and for this reason, tapes can sometimes reveal what simply talking can't. Even more valuable than watching the couples having sex (or not, which was more often the case) was observing how they argued, how they greeted and treated each other at the end of a long day, how supportive they were, who did the housework, who didn't. Whether they snuggled and cuddled after sex or migrated to opposite ends of the bed. When we asked each person how they thought they behaved in these situations, their answers differed dramatically from what actually happened. After seeing real 'evidence' on tape, this alone was sometimes enough incentive for them to face up to the issues they'd been avoiding.

So why I was sitting there watching couples have sex wasn't the issue, it was knowing I had to meet the people afterwards which had me feeling flustered. It's not often you meet someone knowing what they look like naked or what their 'orgasm face' looks like. I felt a bit guilty, like I'd rifled through someone's medicine cabinet while I nipped to the bathroom during a dinner party. Except amplify that 500 times. You can't help but look at people differently once you've seen them 'do it'. Cast your mind back to university, when you'd hear your flatmate groan through paper thin walls and have trouble meeting their eyes as you passed the cornflakes their way the next day. It's slightly surreal shaking someone's hand when you know exactly where it's been (and what it did while it was there). Gingerly placing yourself on a sofa knowing, a mere few hours earlier, the woman offering you a cup of tea was being given oral sex in the exact place you're sitting by the man standing by the mantelpiece. As much as I tried desperately to stay in the moment, images of plunging tongues, bobbing breasts and pumping bottoms whirled in my head. And the whole time I was painfully aware that if I felt strange, imagine how the couples felt, having – quite literally – exposed themselves. What they did was incredibly brave and everyone involved in the project wanted to make sure they were treated with respect; their issues approached sensitively. Despite the normality of the situation, with them offering us cups of tea and us all chatting about the weather, at the back of everyone's mind was the knowledge that pretty soon, 'Could you pass the biscuits?' was going to become, 'So, how's the tongue pressure on your clitoris when your partner gives you oral sex?' It wasn't easy for anyone – but the results made up for any embarrassing moments.

One of the main aims of *The Sex Inspectors* – the TV show and the book – is to reassure people that it's okay not to be the best lover in the world. It's normal not to want sex all the time, not to have an orgasm each time, not to make the earth move. We also hope to dispel the many myths surrounding sex and offer some practical, useful solutions for common problems. Forty per cent of Brits are dissatisfied with their sex lives, there's a fifty per cent divorce rate with roughly the same number admitting to infidelity within a long-term relationship. In an ideal world, we'd all dutifully trot off to see a sex therapist or psychologist to get some help and advice, the same way we go to the doctor for other aches and pains. But as much as it's becoming less of a taboo to 'see someone' and lots of people are very sensibly seeking professional help, others don't and won't because that would mean admitting something really is wrong and that wouldn't do at all. For those people, it could be far less threatening to watch a programme or read a book about sex, especially if it's packaged in an entertaining format, and pick up a few tips that way.

The Sex Inspectors Masterclass is a book about real sex, for real people. One of the things our viewers liked most about the show was they got to see sex as it really is – messy, squidgy and gloriously sweaty. There's something wonderfully reassuring about watching two people make love who don't look perfect (like they do in the movies) and aren't gyrating, moaning and orgasming all over the place (like they do in porn). Just like the TV show, all the tips, tricks and techniques you'll find here are real-life, tried-and-tested. They worked for us, they've worked for our friends – they might just work for you.

One thing I can guarantee – you'll have lots of fun trying them out!

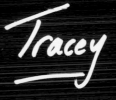

how good are you in bed?

Unfortunately, you can't ask your partner. That's like asking him if those jeans make you look fat – he knows he's going to be sleeping on the couch if he gives the wrong answer. So you're going to have to figure it out yourself. And what better way to do it than with a *Sex Inspectors Masterclass* Quiz? Take it and find out if you're boring in bed or sensational in the sack!

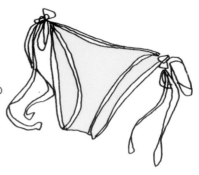

What's considered the 'Male G-spot?'

a The frenulum

b The prostate

c The glans

Where is the 'Male G-spot?'

a A couple of inches inside the anus towards the navel

b A couple of inches inside the urethra towards the bladder

c The thin tissue underneath the point where the coronal ridge meets

The main source of a man's orgasmic pleasure is:

a Ejaculation

b Release of semen

c Pelvic floor muscle contractions

The two most important actions in giving manual or oral stimulation are:

a Pressure and force

b Rubbing and lubrication

c Speed and friction

You can delay a man's orgasm by:

a Becoming more passive

b Slowing down the speed of his thrusts

c Gently tugging his scrotum sack away from his body

You can help your man achieve stronger erections and more powerful orgasms by:

a Trying to climax together

b Doing pelvic floor muscle exercises together

c Doing intimacy building exercises together

The most important combination for performing mind-blowing oral sex on a man is:

a Making sure you're in a comfortable position and taking him in as deep as possible

b Generating lots of saliva and using your hand as an extension of your mouth

c Using personal lubrication and recreating his thrusting motions

For her

Two of the most neglected pleasure zones in a man are:
a The perineum and anus
b The nipples and earlobes
c The scrotum and shaft

After sex, most men want to roll over and go to sleep because:
a They're not that interested in talking afterwards
b They got their cuddles during sex
c Sex depletes energy-producing glycogen from their muscles

Pushing a finger upwards on the perineum will press on what pleasure gland?
a The bladder
b The seminal vesicle
c The prostate

When your man is about to orgasm you should:
a Keep doing what you're doing
b Keep doing what you're doing but speed it up and apply more friction
c Keep doing what you're doing but slow it up and ease the friction.

The best way to find out what your man likes in bed is to:
a Try different things and gauge his reaction
b Wait for him to tell you
c Ask him

To prevent alcohol from ruining your man's performance in bed you should stop him from drinking the:
a Third pint of beer
b Fourth
c Fifth

The best thing you can do to turn your man on in bed is to:
a Be passive and let him take charge
b Be active and take charge
c Respond vocally and physically to what turns you on

The most popular oral sex:
a Starts slowly and builds to a crescendo
b Starts quickly and slows to a crawl
c Starts by deep-throating

1–20

GIRL, WE GOTTA TALK. If things don't improve your partner is going to start calling his mates while he's making love to you. Put yourself on a DIY program. Start by memorizing this book and go from there.

21–41

NOT BAD. But do you really want your partner describing you as 'Not bad in bed?' Time to ditch the half that's not working and work on the half that is. Ask your partner what he'd like and how he'd like it. You'll go from being a Ms Satisfaction to a Sultry Seductress.

42–61

WOW! The sex you're having is so hot you're probably setting off fire alarms. Your partner is one lucky guy. Congratulations!

SCORE! SCORE! SCORE! SCORE! SCORE! SCORE! SCORE!

1. **a** 0, **b** 3, **c** 0	6. **a** 0, **b** 3, **c** 0	11. **a** 2, **b** 3, **c** 0
2. **a** 3, **b** 0, **c** 0	7. **a** 0, **b** 3, **c** 1	12. **a** 2, **b** 0, **c** 3
3. **a** 0, **b** 0, **c** 3	8. **a** 3, **b** 1, **c** 2	13. **a** 3, **b** 0, **c** 0
4. **a** 1, **b** 1, **c** 3	9. **a** 1, **b** 1, **c** 3	14. **a** 1, **b** 1, **c** 3
5. **a** 0, **b** 0, **c** 3	10. **a** 1, **b** 1, **c** 3	15. **a** 3, **b** 0, **c** 0

how good are you in bed?

Anyone can be good in bed – looks don't matter, money doesn't matter and even genital size isn't important. What you do need to become a fully fledged 'sexpert', however, is a good, working knowledge of your lover's sexual response system.

Test your sexual prowess by answering the following:

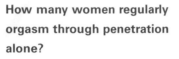

For him

How many women regularly orgasm through penetration alone?
a 80 per cent
b 65 per cent
c 30 per cent

The female G-spot, if indeed there is one, is situated:
a About two inches inside the vagina, on the front wall
b Adjacent to the clitoris
c Just below the vaginal opening

How many women insert a vibrator while masturbating?
a 70 per cent
b 90 per cent
c 15 per cent

The surest way to bring a woman to orgasm is by:
a Giving her oral sex
b Intercourse but with added clitoral stimulation
c By using your hand

The best intercourse position to hit the sensitive front vaginal wall and up her chances of orgasm is:
a Man on top
b Woman on top or rear-entry
c Missionary with her legs on his shoulders

The most accurate way to tell if a woman really has had an orgasm is:
a She'll make lots of noise, then go quiet
b A red rash fleetingly appears on her chest and her clitoris is sensitive to touch immediately afterward
c She'll appear satisfied and stop wanting to have sex

The difference between a male and female orgasm is:
a There is no difference - they are both the same
b Hers tend to be less frequent but last about three times as long
c His is stronger and more intense

The average woman needs at least how much foreplay before being ready for sex:

a Five minutes
b Ten minutes
c Twenty minutes

You've got an extra large penis. To make sex most comfortable for her, the trick is to:

a Spend lots of time on foreplay and use lubricant
b Choose a position which doesn't allow deep penetration
c All of the above

Women most often reach orgasm:

a With their partner
b Through masturbation
c Through oral sex

In general, women have less frequent and less explicit fantasies than men:

a True
b False

The most commonly cited reason for women faking orgasm is:

a I don't want to hurt his feelings
b I want to get sex over with
c I want him to think he's a great lover

The position most women enjoy oral sex in is:

a To have a sixty-niner – both doing it to each other at the same time
b Her lying on her back, pelvis tilted up with a pillow beneath her bottom
c Her straddled over his face

Most women enjoy oral sex which is:

a Done hard, with fast tongue movements
b Varied with lots of different tongue manoeuvres
c Gentle and wet with consistent rhythm

A woman's sex drive is hormonally at its highest:

a Mid cycle when she's ovulating
b During her period
c Immediately after her period

SCORE! SCORE! SCORE! SCORE! SCORE! SCORE! SCORE!

1. **a** 0, **b** 3, **c** 3	6. **a** 1, **b** 3, **c** 0	11. **a** 0, **b** 3
2. **a** 3, **b** 0, **c** 0	7. **a** 0, **b** 3, **c** 0	12. **a** 3, **b** 2, **c** 1
3. **a** 0, **b** 0, **c** 3	8. **a** 0, **b** 0, **c** 3	13. **a** 0, **b** 3, **c** 2
4. **a** 3, **b** 2, **c** 1	9. **a** 2, **b** 1, **c** 3	14. **a** 0, **b** 0, **c** 3
5. **a** 0, **b** 3, **c** 2	10. **a** 0, **b** 3, **c** 2	15. **a** 3, **b** 1, **c** 0

1–20

NOT GREAT Your sexual knowledge is limited and while what works for Mary doesn't necessarily work for Jane, women have all basically got the same hotspots. It's high time you started exploring more, top to toe!

21–41

YOU'RE ABOUT AVERAGE You've got a good, basic working knowledge of her body – but it could be improved. Take a tour around her body, not just the good bits, and ask for a running commentary of what feels hot – or not.

42–61

GO TO THE TOP OF THE CLASS Congratulations! Your knowledge is impressive and you've probably mastered good technique. Score even higher if you talk openly and honestly about sex and make her feel good both in and out of bed.

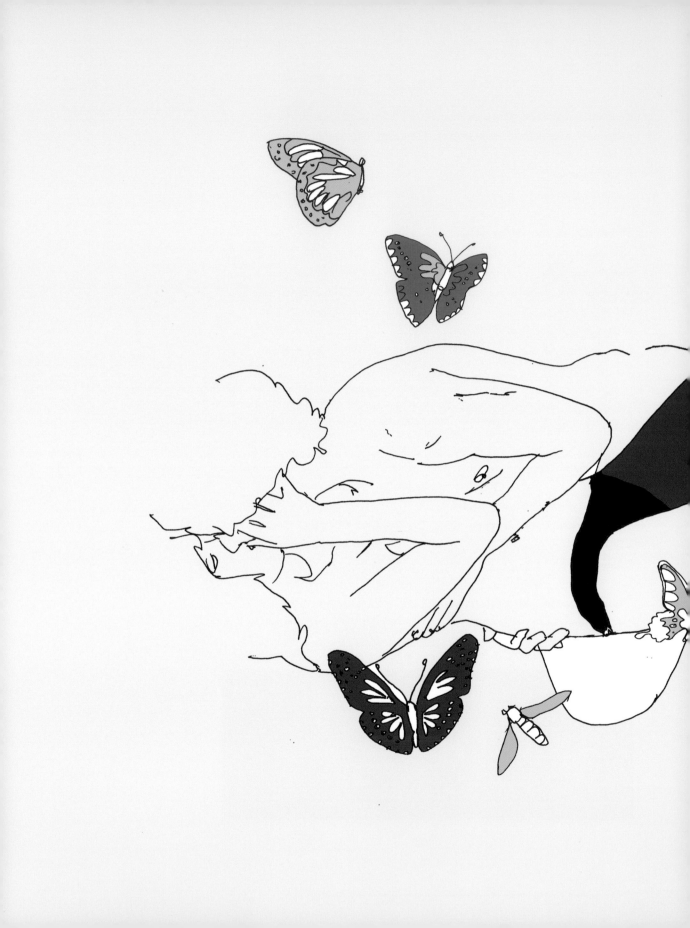

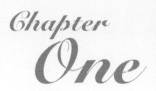

the birds and the bees

Getting a better sex life by getting to know your own body

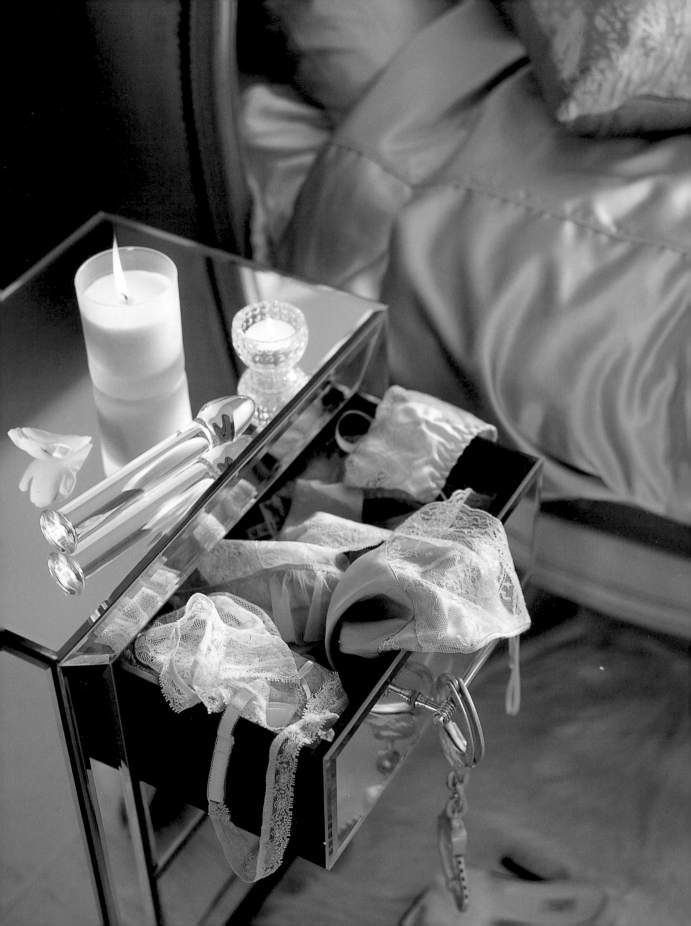

JUST LIKE YOU CAN'T BUILD A BETTER VOCABULARY without knowing the difference between a vowel and a consonant, you can't build a better sex life unless you know the difference between a cervix and a clitoris.

Understanding your sexual system will improve your love life because if you know what's going on you'll know how to make it better. For instance, if you know that muscle contractions are the main source of orgasmic pleasure, then you can find out which muscles to exercise to make those orgasms more powerful. If you know that the 'plateau' stage is where most sexual activity takes place, then knowing how to stay there will help you last longer in bed.

Being aware of your body can help you determine when and if you should go to a doctor and what to ask him or her when you get there. It'll also help you understand their answers better. Better yet, it can alleviate the embarrassment you might have about your genitals. It helps to know you're not the only one with a curved penis or labia minora that hang a bit longer than the labia majora.

Knowledge can also heal sexual embarrassment by throwing daylight on the myths that darken your self-esteem. Are you feeling inadequate about the size of your penis because you 'know' the average is six inches? Well, it isn't. Are you feeling 'abnormal' because you're one of the few women who can't orgasm through penetration? Well, you're not. Knowledge has the power to educate, illuminate and enlighten. So onward! Or inward! Or outward!

two of a kind

THE MOST ASTOUNDING THING ABOUT MEN and women is that despite how differently we look, our bodies are mirror images of each other. Males and females start out as identical blobs of tissue when the sperm enters the egg. Even with ultrasound, you can't tell the difference between male and female babies until the fifteenth week of pregnancy.

The same tissue that turns into ovaries in women turns into testicles for men. The same tissue that forms vaginal lips in women forms scrotal sacs in men. The same tissue that turns into a penis in men turns into a clitoris for women. In fact, both the penis and clitoris have a glans and a shaft and become engorged with blood when sexually stimulated. So much for penis envy.

Although there are major differences in the way we experience sex, the journey is remarkably similar. Almost all men and women go through a four-step sexual response cycle. (Five if your partner lets you roll over and sleep.)

AROUSAL Sex starts with seeing, thinking, touching, smelling or fantasizing about something or someone that turns you on. A new Mercedes, maybe. A woman who makes the sky long for the blue of her eyes, or a guy who makes wilted flowers stand to attention when he walks by. Extra blood starts pumping to key areas of your body – your genitals, lips, earlobes and other parts. Men get an erection when the two large cylinders of spongy tissue in their penis fill with blood. These cylinders are covered by a tough fibrous sheath and when they fill up with blood they push against this sheath, much the way pumping air into a tyre pushes against its rubber walls, creating something strong enough to take a ride on. The muscles in the scrotum contract, moving the testicles up towards your pelvis.

If you think men swell up like a storm, watch the hurricane whipping up in women: the vaginal walls secrete a watery fluid, moistening all of the external genitals. The outer vaginal lips swell and open up while the inner lips become thicker and longer. The vagina expands, the clitoris enlarges, and the nipples harden. The areolae around them swell and darken. The uterus and cervix engorge and lift towards the pelvis. A fine skin rash or 'sex flush' develops on the chest, back and abdomen.

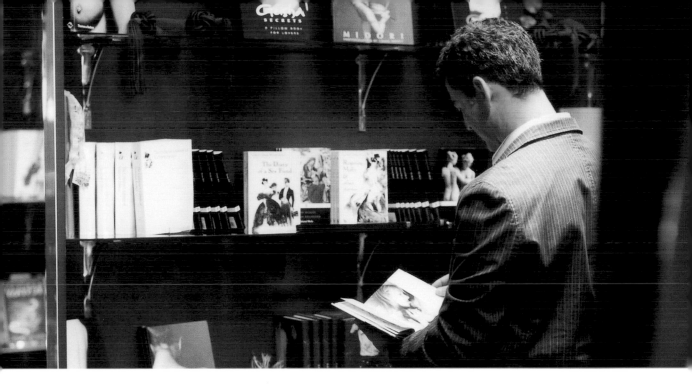

Pleasure fluctuates with highs and lows ... it's perfectly natural for erections to wax and wane

PLATEAU In this stage, everything in both sexes increasingly swells, lifts and darkens. The inner vagina expands up to three times its normal diameter, but the lower third of the vagina doesn't. It decreases, creating a constriction that grips the penis during penetration. The result? A pulling of the labia and clitoral hood during thrusting, giving everyone involved a well-deserved smile. At any rate, you're kissing, you're touching, you're having a ball. Pleasure fluctuates with highs and lows but never ends. It's perfectly natural for erections to wax and wane in the plateau stage. For instance, you may lose your erection while going down on a woman even though you love doing it. No worries. All it means is that giving oral sex doesn't keep you hard. You'll get it back. In women, the clitoris says 'yes, yes' and 'no, no' at the same time because it's experiencing fear and excitement simultaneously. The super-sensitive organ may protect itself from direct stimulation by retreating under the clitoral hood. It may mean your partner should back off. Rough handling of 8,000 nerve endings in an area less than an inch in size screams 'SENSORY OVERLOAD', so proceed with caution.

The plateau stage is where most of the manual, oral and penetrative sex happens. Most people want to establish residency here because it just feels too good to leave.

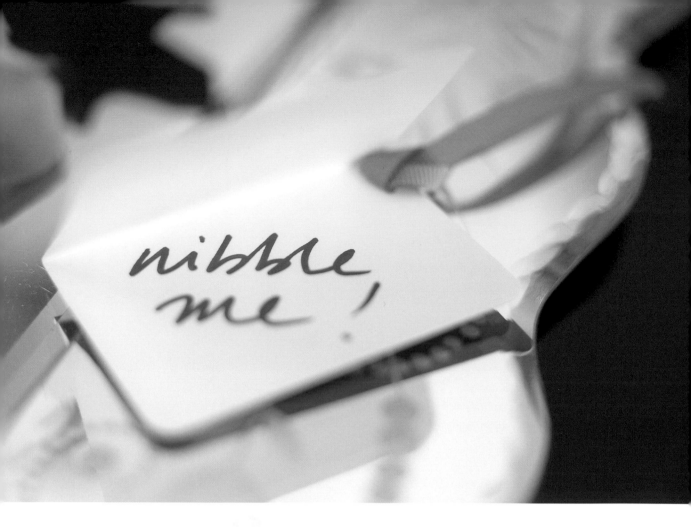

ORGASM As you advance from the plateau stage the pleasure peaks and men start gasping toward 'ejaculatory inevitability' (the point where nothing is going to stop your orgasm – not even your mum walking in on you). Here's what happens: everything starts to contract. Your testicles ascend until they press against the wall of the pelvis. The prostate, seminal vesicles and vas deferens squeeze themselves silly, pouring their sperm and seminal fluid like bartenders who can't keep up with the orders. The head of the penis becomes deep purple while the shaft increasingly stiffens. Breathing, blood pressure and heartbeat increase as the total-body response to ejaculation takes over. Involuntary spasms in the legs, feet, toes, stomach, arms and back can take over. The pelvic muscles go through a series of rhythmic contractions, ejaculating semen through the urethra as a series of spurts. And that, in a nutshell, is how every other thought that men may have had during the day ends at night.

Again, the sexual storms in men look like spring showers compared to the ones in women. The vagina's inner lips go from bright pink to dark red. Mounting tension triggers an initial spasm and then a series of muscle contractions around the lower third of the vagina. Simultaneously, rhythmic spasms ripple down from the uterus to the cervix. Pulse, breathing, blood pressure and skin flushes peak, while contractions in different muscle groups make the face contort, the spine arch, the abdomen tighten, the buttocks squeeze, the hands clench, the toes curl and the ankles straighten. Glands in the vagina continue to secrete clear fluid, making the entire vulva feel wet during orgasm. Muscles in the uterus and vagina contract, lasting from four to fifteen seconds or more – even up to a minute! Muscle spasms tend to occur in sequences of just under a second. Unlike men, orgasm doesn't necessarily mean the end of sex. Women can almost immediately have a second or third or twelfth orgasm, one after the other.

RESOLUTION

You know how everything contracts during orgasm? The opposite happens during the resolution phase. It's as if your body got shot to the moon and now it's gravity's turn to teach you a lesson. In men, the blood flows out of the penis and the scrotum descends. Pulse, breathing and blood pressure rates return to normal. In women, the sex flush disappears and is often replaced with a film of perspiration. The clitoris returns to its normal size and position and the vagina shrinks to its resting length and diameter. The uterus and cervix descend from the pelvic ceiling. While everything slides down, relaxes or shrinks, the cervical canal doesn't. It dilates, probably to make it easier for the sperm to do the backstroke into the uterus. Women can have another go at sex right away. Men usually can't, they go through a refractory period in which they can't get erect (for some a minute or two; for others a day or two and for most, somewhere in between). Just because women can have sex again right away doesn't mean they want to. Many find their vulva, particularly the clitoris, becomes too sensitive.

At any rate, the tension released by orgasm feels exquisite to both men and women. That's why the first letter in orgasm should be spelled 'ohh'.

Now, united you may have stood (or lain), but divided you shall fall: Women tend to be more alert after orgasm while men become somewhat catatonic. Oxytocin, the 'cuddle chemical', tends to flood women after sex, while men get drained of glycogen, a vital source for energy. And that's why women want to bond after sex and men want to snore.

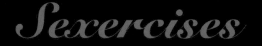

Sexercises

Both men and women can improve the intensity of their orgasms by strengthening the pelvic floor muscles. Remember, the main source of an orgasm's pleasure is the release of tension the muscle contractions provide. Strengthen the muscles and you strengthen the orgasms. In women, these exercises can also tighten the vaginal opening and improve bladder control (a common problem after giving birth). In men, the exercises can improve the strength of erections (by expanding blood flow to the penis) and help you last longer by giving you more control of your ejaculations. Named after the doctor who invented them, 'Kegels' stretch and strengthen the pelvic muscles crucial to sexual functioning. Relaxation between the contractions is key, especially for men who want to last longer in bed. If you learn how to relax the pelvic muscles (which spasm during orgasm) you can delay your ejaculations. Do Kegels for a minimum of six weeks. Like going to the gym, you're not going to see immediate results.

Here's a step-by-step guide on how to do them:

● **LOCATE YOUR PELVIC MUSCLES** by stopping the flow of urine midstream.

● **CONTRACT THE PELVIC MUSCLES** hard for a second or two and then release them. Do it ten times in a row, three times a day. Then gradually increase the number of contractions so that by the end of six weeks, you're doing about ten contractions, twenty times a day.

● **VARY THE EXERCISES.** Try 'The Flutter' (tighten and let go quickly) and the 'Pinch and Hold' (tighten and don't let go till you count to fifteen).

● **VARY THE POSITIONS.** Don't do them all while sitting or standing. Try Kegeling while lying on your back or side or while squatting. Different positions tone the muscle quicker.

● **ADD 'WEIGHT TRAINING'.** Men can place a towel on their erect penis and move it up and down. See how many towels you can lift. You want more bragging rights? Do them with wet towels.

● **KEGEL EVERYWHERE.** Watching TV, talking on the phone, driving your car, reading this book, you can do them anywhere at any time. Even when you're making love. Men can have their partner hold a finger about an inch above your erect penis and flex hard enough to touch it ten times in a row. Women can contract the muscles when your partner is inside you. It'll feel like his penis is getting massaged.

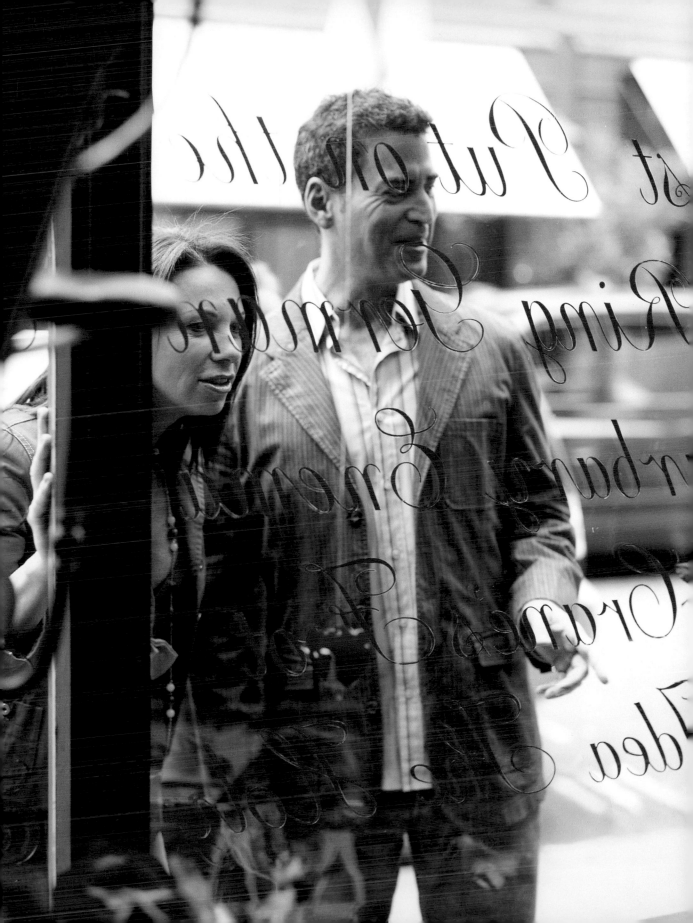

vive la difference!

Men orgasm more often, but women have far more intense experiences

NOW THAT WE KNOW HOW MEN AND WOMEN are alike, let's take a look at how much we're not. At the risk of stating the obvious, men's genitals are external, while women's are not. For the most part, anyway. It's friction through the vagina that gives men orgasms. It's friction on the clitoris that gives women theirs. The head of a man's penis has about 4,000 nerve endings; the much smaller clitoris has about 8,000. Men can reach orgasm in two or three minutes; women usually need ten to twenty minutes. Men have a refractory period in which most can't get aroused; women don't. Males reach the height of their orgasmic power at around age fifteen; women at twenty-nine. Male climaxes last for a few seconds (average is 5), while female orgasms can last three times longer (on average 15). Almost all men orgasm during sex, while less than half of women do. Men orgasm more often, but women have far more intense experiences.

It is the great paradox of sex that men and women are so fundamentally similar yet so functionally different. We may be cut from the same cloth, but we wear entirely different clothes. Let's take a closer look at the differences between the sexes.

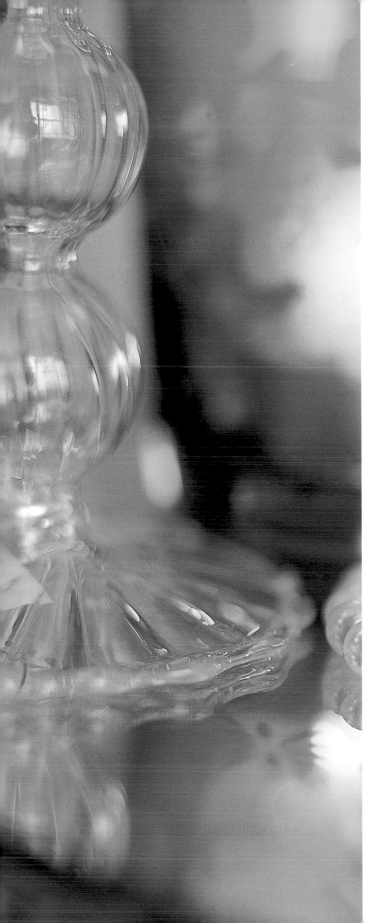

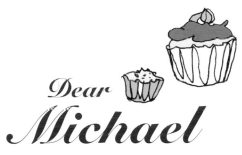

Dear *Michael*

MY WIFE AND I WANT TO TRY FANTASY
AND ROLE PLAY BUT WE DON'T KNOW
HOW TO START AND DON'T EVEN HAVE
A CLEAR IDEA OF OUR OWN FANTASIES.
HOW CAN WE FORMALIZE OUR
FANTASIES IN A WAY THAT WE CAN
ACT THEM OUT?

Start by asking yourself how you want to feel or how you want people to react to you. Do you want them to adore you? Hate you? That's your starting point. Then imagine what type of person epitomizes that feeling to you, ie the role your partner will need to play. Be warned that you may not share each other's fantasies, but you can take turns, so she could be the supporting actress in your fantasy and the star in her own! And it's a good idea to try swapping roles, playing one may give you ideas about the other. Other aspects to consider are location, costumes and music, all of which will make your fantasy seem more real. And remember that one of you has to take control of the fantasy. If one of you is going to strip, somebody's got to decide how. I say if it's your fantasy then you be the boss. Finally, being in character may give you the confidence to try new things and expand your sexual horizons. Go for it!

the birds and the bees

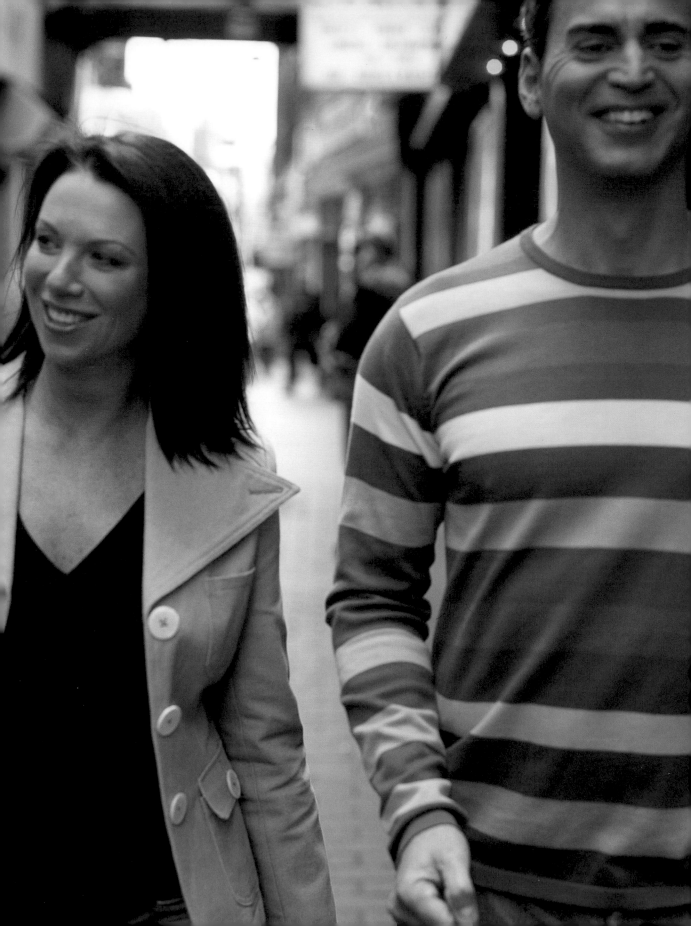

Men's Bits

MEET YOUR DECISION MAKER

The penis has a head (glans) with a much higher concentration of nerve endings than the shaft. The glans has a coronal ridge separating it from the shaft (the outer edge of the 'helmet'). On the underside of the penis there's a small triangular region where a thin strip of skin called the frenulum attaches to the glans. Both the coronal ridge and the frenulum are highly sensitive. If it's true that men think with their penis, then this is the command centre.

HEADS UP!

About ninety-five per cent of men in the UK are uncircumcised. The good news for those ninety-five per cent is that uncircumcised penises are more sensitive. They're protected from rubbing, scratching and scraping against clothing.

However, there are arguments for and against and uncircumcised men do have to be more conscientious about cleaning their penis than their circumcised counterparts. That's because smegma, a cheesy secretion, can form under the foreskin unless it's cleaned daily. While clinical studies show it has anti-bacterial and anti-viral properties, it also has anti-women properties.

Men are far more obsessed with the size of their penis than women are

MIND THE GAP

There's a small strip of skin bridging the gap between your scrotum and anus. It's called the perineum and it's highly sensitive to the touch because it's packed with nerve endings. Sure, the tube can take you directly to your destination, but minding the gap will make the journey so much more pleasant. Ask your partner to stroke it gently or press one or two fingers upwards, where the hyper-sensitive prostate resides.

THE PENIS: SIZING IT UP

Men are far more obsessed with the size of their penis than women are. In survey after survey women don't even rank it in the top five. So if it generally doesn't matter to women, why does it matter so much to men?

First, because we have a 'bigger is better' mentality. It's called 'Male Maths': Size + Size= Status on Stilts. That's why men love bigger cars, bigger biceps, bigger wallets, bigger everything.

Secondly, the only time heterosexual men see other erect penises is when they're watching porn, where every penis needs its own space in the car park. So they have a completely unrealistic view of what a 'normal' sized erect penis looks like.

Thirdly, many men still believe that most women orgasm through penetration. So the more you have to penetrate her with the more sexually satisfied she'll be, right? Wrong. Seventy-eighty per cent of women orgasm through stimulation of the clitoris, which is best done by a talented hand or a lubricated tongue. Preferably both.

'IT'S NOT VERY BIG BUT I'M PROUD OF EVERY FOOT'

MILKING IT FOR ALL IT'S WORTH

What's in the milky white stuff anyway? For the most part, semen is made of sugar, water, enzymes, protein, zinc and citric and ascorbic acid (Vitamin C). There's not enough of anything in it to cause harm or good. There's a wide variety of consistency and viscosity in semen, but for the most part it comes out white and then turns clear. Here's why: the two glands that make up most of the liquid in semen are at odds with each other. The seminal vesicle contains sugars and proteins that cause semen to coagulate, turning it white. But fluid from the prostate gland contains enzymes that break down that coagulation. So basically, your ejaculate doesn't know whether it's coming or going. So it does both. It coagulates as soon as it leaves your penis, then immediately goes into 'liquefaction'.

Pop quiz

DOES PENIS SIZE MATTER TO WOMEN?

A survey in *The Kinsey Institute New Report on Sex* asked women which physical characteristics turned them on the most:

a. Penis size
b. Firm muscle tone
c. Well-groomed hair
d. Clear complexion
e. White teeth

Penis size ranked last. Bottom line: you'd attract more women by combing your hair and brushing your teeth than by growing your penis.

Despite all the evidence, man's fixation with the size of the prize goes unabated. And unmeasured. So if you're going to obsess, at least know the benchmarks. Here's what the latest studies show:

● Average length when erect: 5.1 inches
● Average girth when erect: 4.8 inches
● Average length when flaccid: 3.5 inches

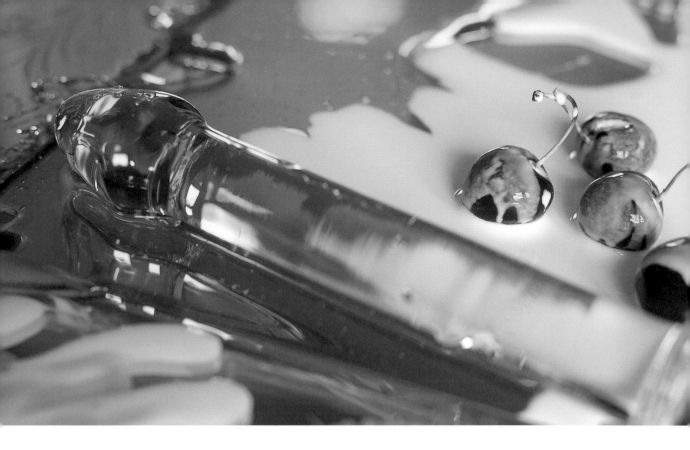

A DROP IN THE BUCKET

Ever notice whenever you get an erection that several drops of clear liquid ooze out of your penis? It's called 'Pre-ejaculatory fluid'. About thirty per cent of men have it. Sexual excitement squeezes the prostate and seminal vesicles and forces the fluid up (ranging from a drop to several drops). What's the point of the drops? They serve as a built-in reservoir of lubrication. They also neutralize acid in the urethra from residual urine, keeping sperm safe for their journey to Eggland.

AFTER THE FACT

● Only two per cent of semen is actually made up of sperm (that's why men don't notice any difference in semen volume after they get vasectomies).

● About five per cent of women are allergic to semen.

● The average man ejaculates about a teaspoonful of semen.

● The average ejaculation has 12 calories.

● There is enough sperm in pre-ejaculate to impregnate women.

That's why 'pulling out' just before you ejaculate doesn't always work.

The right way to measure your penis

● Use a cloth measuring tape, not a straight-edged ruler.

● Measure to the nearest half-centimetre, not the nearest half-foot.

● Measure as soon as you undress. The temperature of the room will affect your length and girth. Why miss a millimetre if you don't have to?

● Do not measure the side of the penis connected to the scrotum. Why? Well, where would you stop? That's a sneaky way to add an inch or two. Nice try. Measure the side of the penis facing your stomach. It'll eliminate man's mapmaker's mentality. You know, the one that says, 'one inch = one mile.'

● Place the measuring tape at the junction of skin between the lower belly and the base of your penis. Then unroll it to the top.

● Read it and weep.

Quickie questions

● WHY IS MY PENIS DARKER THAN THE REST OF MY BODY? It's part of the sexual maturation process, but it's also because during puberty you discover someone you'll shake hands with for the rest of your life. Over the years, masturbation darkens the skin.

● WHY IS THERE A LINE GOING DOWN MY PENIS AND TESTICLES? All men have it. It's a sort of 'seam' on the underside of the penis. It forms when the foetus is in the uterus. In women, the seam becomes the vagina's inner lips. In men, the seam encloses the urethra along the length of the penis.

PLAY BALL!

The scrotum is the sack that holds the testicles, which produce sperm and testosterone, the jet fuel for erections. The muscles in the scrotum are affected by temperature. When it's warm, the muscles pull out a deckchair and start sunning themselves, making the scrotum and testicles hang lower. When it's cold the muscles fold up the deckchair and bring the boys in for some hot tea. One testicle hangs lower than the other in eighty-five per cent of men. And it's usually the left one. Testicles seem to have a life of their own. Next time you're lying in bed naked, look without touching them. Notice how they're moving by themselves? It's called 'testicular circulation' – blood coursing throughout the scrotum.

Women's Bits

'What you don't know about women is a lot'

Olympia Dukakis said that to a man in the movie *Moonstruck*, but it could just as easily be applied to women. Part of the reason so many women are in the dark about their parts is that their parts are in the dark. Unlike men, whose genitals stick out so much they cast puppet shadows on the wall, women's bits are mostly internal. Men look, touch and examine their genitals all the time, so we're much more familiar with our genitals than women are with theirs. It's time to put that to an end.

IT'S NOT A STYLISH SWEDISH CAR BUT HERE ARE THE KEYS TO YOUR VULVA

A woman's entire collection of genitals, from the vagina to the uterus, is called the vulva. To really understand your anatomy we'll need some investigatory tools – a mirror, a lamp and a door, behind which you can leave all your inhibitions.

Sit on the floor, bend your knees and spread them apart. Use the mirror and the lamp. Don't be shy. At first, the only thing you'll see between your legs is a vertical slit between two plump 'lips' (labia majora). Trace your fingers along the lips. At the back they end in a small stretch of muscle in front of your anus (the perineum). At the front they end at the pubic mound, directly south of your navel. This pad of fat protects your pubic bone when you're making love or leaning too far forward on your bike.

Now, part the outer lips with your fingers and you'll see the inner lips (labia minora) inside. Follow them forwards. The fold where they meet is the hood covering the clitoris. Pull it back and you'll feel a bump of tissue about the size of a large pea. Congratulations, you've reached Ground Zero of Pleasure Central. Use lubricant and press

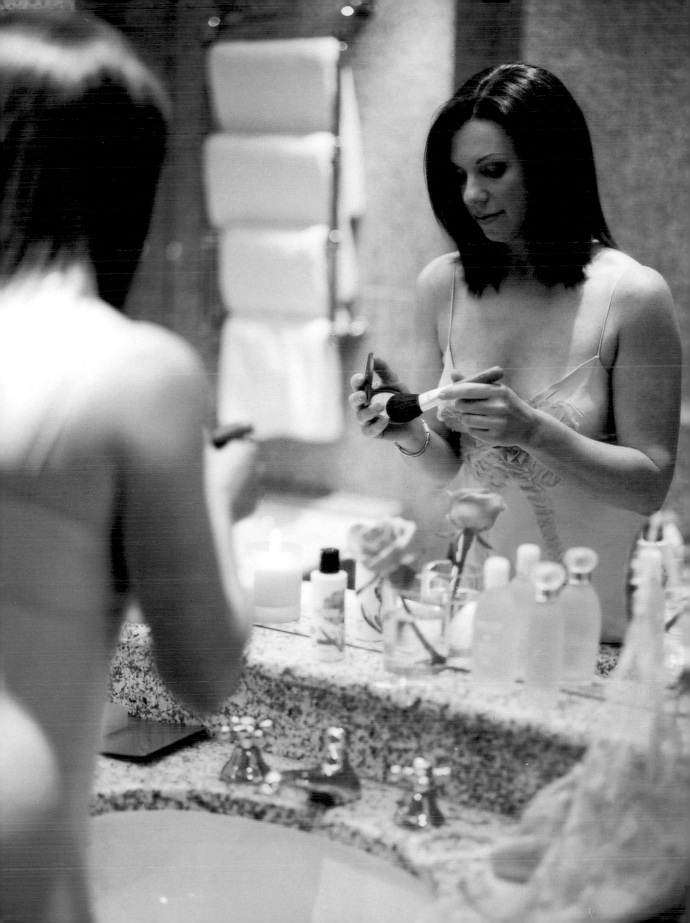

gently in a circular motion around the edges of the clitoris and you'll feel a pleasant stirring. Note the clitoris becomes firmer and pokes out of its hood, much the way the head of an uncircumcised penis pokes out of its foreskin. There's a rubbery rod extending a few inches back into your body to the pubic bone. That's the clitoral shaft. The clitoral glans (the part that peeks out from the hood) is about a quarter-inch in diameter. Does it feel better if you press above it, below or around it? Do you like light pressure, heavy pressure or no pressure? Do you like circled motions, up-and-down strokes or grazing touches? It's important to work this out because if you want your partner to send you to the moon, you're going to have to show him how to find the launch button.

TWIN PEAKS

Breasts are not exactly identical twins. One is almost always bigger or hangs lower than the other. Just like a man's testicles. Nothing hangs off the body in perfect symmetry. The nipple juts out from the centre of the breast, surrounded by the areola. If you're nursing a baby, the little bumps on the areola secrete a natural body oil

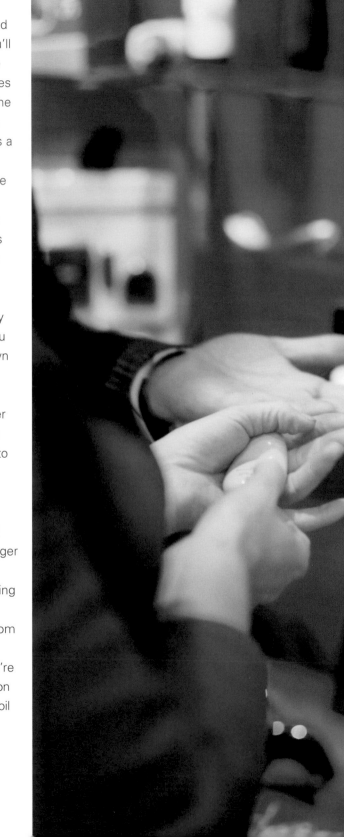

to reduce any friction caused by the baby's sucking motion.

Although men consider breasts double domes of erogenous zones, not all women enjoy having them touched or kissed. Take your hands and do some stimulus testing. What feels best? Gentle touching or stroking or a harder massaging motion? And while your hands are there take the time to take care of your health. Feel around for lumps every month. If you notice any, talk to a doctor.

ASHAMED OF YOUR LABIA?

Lots of women think there's something wrong with their labia minora, especially if they hang further than the labia majora. Relax. There's nothing wrong. Since you rarely see other women's labias, you've compared yourself to oversimplified diagrams showing neat, symmetrical labia. The truth is, there's no such thing as 'normal' labia minora. They are rarely symmetrical, the skin colour ranges from a bright pink to a dark purplish-brown, and the texture can be smooth or wrinkled.

Although men consider breasts the double domes of erogenous zones, not all women enjoy having them touched or kissed

MIRROR, MIRROR ON THE FLOOR, WHERE'S THE PART THAT MAKES ME ROAR?

Insert your fingers into the vaginal opening and you'll notice it's not actually a hole. The sides of the vaginal tunnel touch one another if there isn't a finger, a tampon, a penis or a toy occupying the space.
The vagina is a muscular tube that is, on average, about four inches long. It's situated at an upward angle towards the small of your back, not horizontally toward your tailbone or vertically towards your stomach. Remind your partner: everything goes in easier at an upward angle.
The vagina extends to the cervix, the gateway to your uterus. A penis can't push into the uterus because the entrance is narrower than a drinking straw. If you give birth, though, this gateway will open wide. Very wide. Babies can get out, but penises can't get in. Go figure.

Quickie questions

● WHY DO I FEEL EXTRA SEXY AT CERTAIN TIMES OF THE MONTH?
Some women have an irresistible urge to show their personal appreciation
to every member of Manchester United round about mid cycle.
Oestrogen levels are highest during ovulation, amping up the libido. If
your sex drive doesn't change, that's normal, too. Hormonal changes
affect some more than others.

● IS IT DANGEROUS TO HAVE SEX WHEN I'M MENSTRUATING?
No, not if you don't care about your sheets. Just make sure to remove the
tampon before having sex. Otherwise, the tampon can be pushed in so
far you'll need a doctor to get it out and risk a possible infection. Believe it
or not, having an orgasm is the best way to relieve menstrual cramps.
During menstruation the muscles around the uterus and the intestines contract harder than usual. Orgasms relieve the contractions.

● IS THERE REALLY A G-SPOT AND HOW CAN I FIND IT?
The jury is still out but some still swear the answer is, 'Yes! Yes! Oh God,
yes!' Not all women appear to have this cluster of nerve endings and
glands, though. Here's how to find out if you have one: first, empty your
bladder because in some women, stimulating the G-spot makes them feel
like they have to pee. Squat down and insert a well-lubricated finger into
your vagina (aim for your belly button). Because the G-spot lies flat
against the vaginal wall, you can't feel it until it's aroused, when it'll swell
up. So stimulate yourself in a way that feels good. Did you find a raised,
textured area about the size of a walnut? Well done!

● WHY DOES MY VAGINA MAKE FARTING NOISES AFTER SEX?
Sometimes a vigorous intercourse session can push a little air into the vagina, which is released with the same sound as passing gas. There's no real
way of avoiding it, short of having gentler, kinder sex. If you experience
'vaginal flatulence,' do what guys do. Blame it on the dog.

Oh, Swell

THE CLITORIS IS THE ONLY SEXUAL ORGAN IN THE HUMAN BODY THAT EXISTS STRICTLY FOR PLEASURE. EVERY OTHER SEXUAL ORGAN IN MALES AND FEMALES SERVES A REPRODUCTIVE FUNCTION.

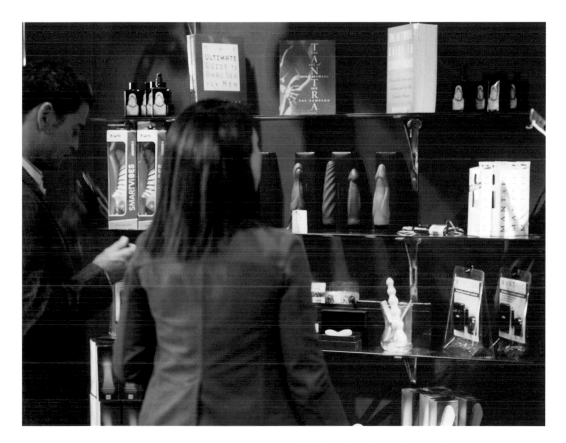

MATHS PROBLEM If the average vagina is four inches long and the average erect penis is 5.1 inches long, what happens when Harry meets Sally? Answer: the vaginal walls stretch to accommodate the difference. Typically, when a woman is aroused, her uterus and cervix will ascend, lengthening the vaginal tube. If Harry's swinging a ten-inch bat, however, Sally might have to call a time out.

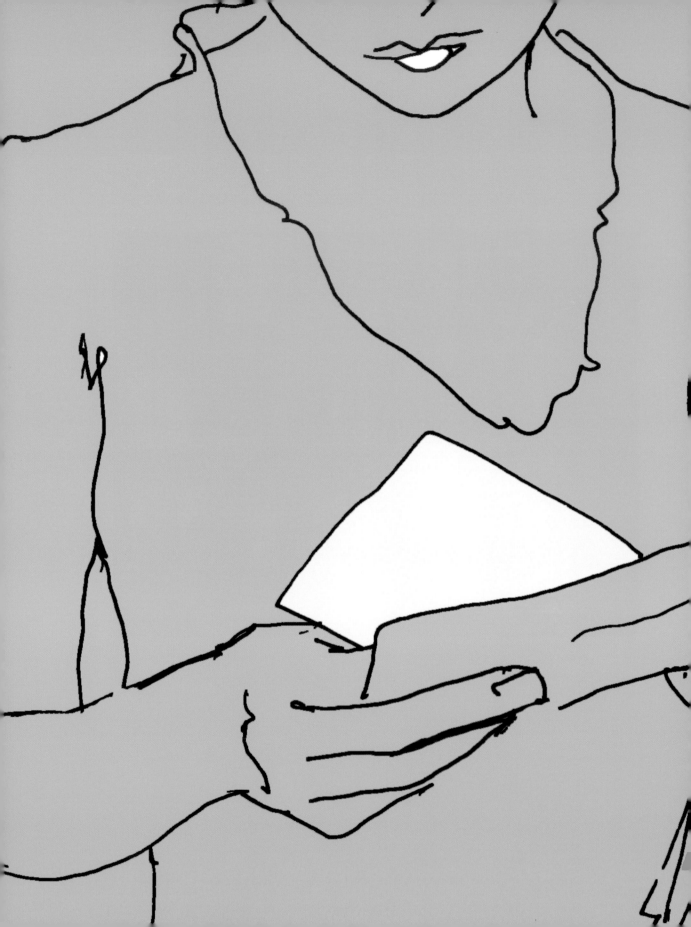

Chapter TWO

clever
communication

No-cringe, ultra-easy ways to
talk to your lover about sex

*S*AYING MANY PEOPLE FIND IT EMBARRASSING to talk about sex is a little like saying most people would prefer not to have all their toes cut off. It's a ridiculous understatement. For some people, discussing sex problems is such taboo territory, they probably would opt for chopped off toes and an extra £100,000 added to their mortgage than admit straight up that, sorry dear, all is not well.

The reason is that sex is shrouded in such mystery and secrecy, it's practically squashed under a pile of dusty old myths. Like the one that says if you love someone, you'll know exactly what to do to please them, without them ever uttering a word of instruction. As well as practising psychic sex, there's a perception that we're born good lovers. No one has to be educated about sex (Goodness me! How vulgar!), you're just supposed to know what a clitoris is and how best to stimulate it, what to do with a frenulum and how to find a G-spot. Where this divine knowledge stems from isn't explained but the end result is that most people's sex lives are a quarter as good as they could be, purely through lack of communication.

Well, we're about to fix that. This chapter tells you how to air your orgasm anxieties, as painlessly as possible. And yes, I know you're squirming at the mere thought of having to 'fess up, but let's make something abundantly clear here, before you decide it's all too difficult and stick your head back in the sand. If your partner's not making you happy in bed, you have four choices:

There's a perception that we're born good lovers

A Telling Test

Can you name the top three places your partner loves to be touched?

Come on, right off the top of your head, without even thinking about it, list off your partner's three hot zones. If you don't know the answer or spend the next few hours struggling to even come up with one or two, your sex life could be in trouble. Let's be honest here: if you don't even know what areas they'd most like stimulated, what chance have you got of being No 1 on the 'Best Lover in their Life' list? Feel incredibly (and justifiably) smug if you can not only name your partner's top three favourite spots but their three second favourites as well. Truly brilliant lovers also realize these zones can change according to mood, time of month, stress levels and how tired/happy/drunk we are. And stroking that secret spot just below her belly button may well make her sigh on thin days, but go anywhere near when she's feeling bloated/full up/in the grips of PMT and you could find yourself unexpectedly a eunuch.

DUMP THEM and find someone else
(an excellent solution if you're only with them for
sex, but unlikely since they're bad at it).

PUT UP WITH IT (and resign yourself to a lifetime
of frustration, resentment and dissatisfaction which
inevitably accompanies putting up with bad sex).

PUT UP WITH IT BUT HAVE SEX ON THE SIDE
(that's called an affair and there's plenty of reasons why that
isn't the answer. See Chapter Eight).

TALK ABOUT IT and suffer half an hour (max!) of possible embarrassment
(and more than likely turn bad sex into mind-blowingly bloody amazing sex!)

So what will it be? Hmmmm? Good! Now we've got that argument out of the way, the rest is easy …

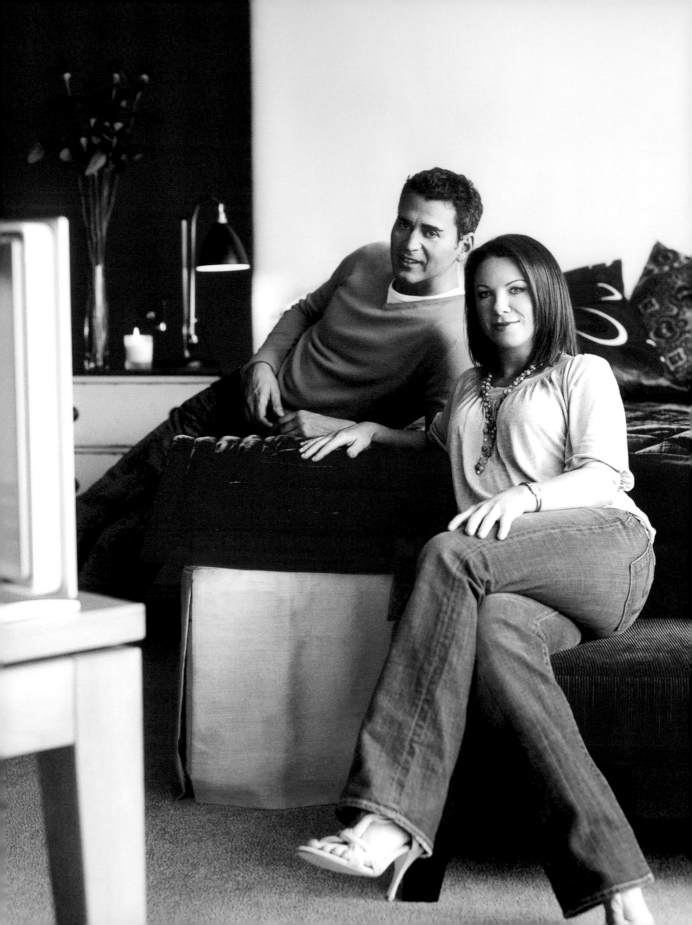

what's happening
outside the bedroom

DURING THE FILMING OF THE SEX INSPECTORS, we watched lots of couples romping about. Truth is, though, Michael and I often learned more about the couple's sex life from how they communicated out of bed than from what they did in it. It makes sense. If you're desperately unhappy in your relationship – forcing yourself to pucker up for a hello kiss and having to hide your joy when being told they're off to attend a week-long conference in Siberia – it's highly unlikely you'll be eagerly grabbing for breasts/bottoms/other bits once under the covers. If you want great sex tonight, treat your partner well today.

Sometimes it's blatantly obvious your relationship's going through a rough patch (the last time you sat at the table together, there were divorce lawyers present). Other times, you think things are okay, but you're not entirely sure. You're happy enough but … are they? Are those congratulatory champagne clinks on anniversaries real or are they putting on a brave face because they don't want to hurt you?

It's in situations like these where body language comes into its own. Forget what they're saying, look at the messages their body is sending you. It takes courage to say, 'Honey, I think we're in one hell of a rut,' and by voicing their unhappiness it suddenly makes it real. This is why their body will often tell you they're unhappy before their words do. See how you and your partner score on the following and if you're not satisfied, it's time for one of those (dreaded but necessary) 'We need to talk' chats.

If you want great sex tonight, treat your partner well today

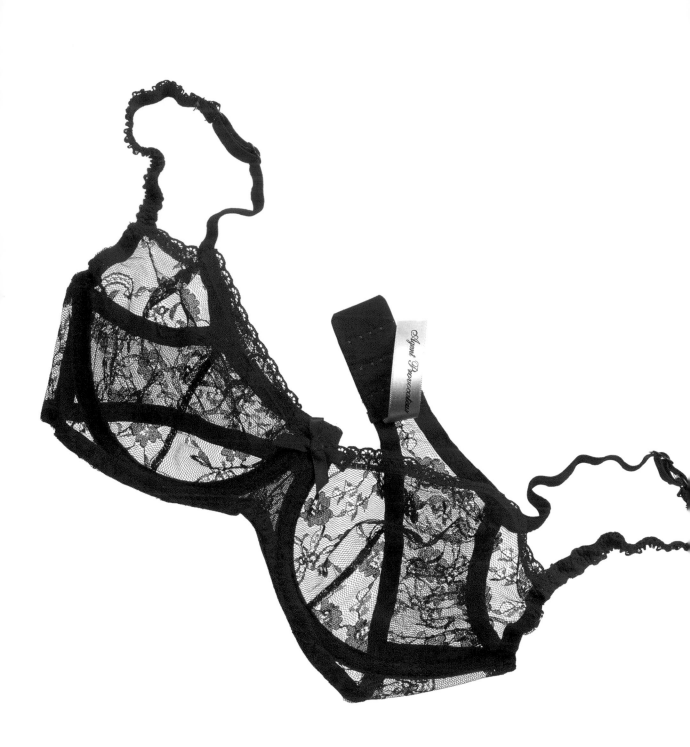

clever communication

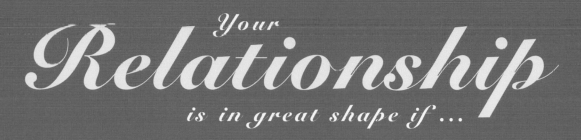

Your Relationship

is in great shape if ...

● **THEY LOOK YOU STRAIGHT IN THE EYE.** Direct eye contact means they have nothing to hide.

● **THEY'LL SIT ON THE SOFA BESIDE YOU,** rather than in a separate chair. Wanting to be physically close during 'relax' time, means the relationship gives them comfort and isn't stressful.

● **YOUR UPPER TORSOS ARE CLOSE WHEN YOU HUG EACH OTHER.** As a general rule, the closer your hearts, the closer you feel emotionally.

● **YOU PRESS PELVISES WHEN YOU HUG.** The closer the hips, the better and more frequent the sex. If you closely connect from your shoulders right through to your knees, you have a perfect balance between great sex and love.

● **THEY TOUCH THEIR FOREHEAD** to yours when you hug or just before you kiss. This is a sign of great trust and affection.

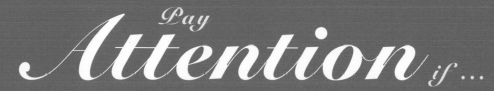

Pay Attention *if ...*

● **THEY STAND FAR APART FROM YOU.** Physical distance usually equates to emotional distance.

● **THE ONLY TIME YOU SEEM TO TOUCH IS WHEN YOU MEET,** say goodbye or have sex. You've lost physical intimacy and turned into friends with benefits.

● **THEY LEAN IN TO KISS YOU HELLO AND GOODBYE** rather than snuggle in and get close.

● **THEY AVOID MEETING YOUR EYES.** They're hiding something (or someone?) or want to avoid acknowledging how bad the relationship has become.

● **THEIR BODY LANGUAGE IS CLOSED.** We use 'closed' body language – trying to put barriers between us and another person – to protect ourselves. If they always seem to fold their arms, hold their drink between you, keep their bag on the shoulder closest to you, cross legs away from you or lean back and away, it's not great news.

clever communication

a portrait of your relationship

Photos provide a telling snapshot of how your relationship was in that moment

PHOTOGRAPHS OF THE TWO OF YOU don't just provide lovely memories of places you've been and people you've seen. They're a rather handy way to see how your relationship and sex life are holding up over time. Photos provide a telling snapshot of how your relationship was in that moment because it captures your body language. By analysing that, you can get a good idea of how you related to each other then and how you relate now.

IF YOU'VE ONLY BEEN TOGETHER A SHORT TIME, grab all your photos and put them in order. Start from when you first got together to the present day. If you've been together for a long time, try to pick one photo to represent each six-month block. Now examine how you stand, sit, kiss and walk together. Compare how close you stood together then to now. How much are you touching? Look at your facial expressions: do you see happiness or resentment? Look at the shoulders: are they back and proud (happy), slumped forward (depressed) or held high (tense)? Is the smile genuine (eyes crinkled, cheeks lifted in balls)? Are your torsos turned towards or away from each other? Run through all the points listed under 'What's happening outside the bedroom?' (page 45) and apply them to the pictures.

IF YOU SUSPECT A SIGNIFICANT EVENT changed the way you feel towards each other, organize the pictures into before and after the situation and repeat the process.

CHOOSE THE PICTURE YOU'RE HAPPIEST WITH – one which demonstrates how you'd like the two of you to be now (congratulations if it was taken yesterday!). Also, find one which reflects your unhappiest period – how you'd least like to be. Put both somewhere handy.

THE NEXT TIME YOU AND YOUR PARTNER ARE CHATTING comfortably, bring out the pictures and show them. Explain the exercise you've done and what you learned from it and use it as a springboard to talk through where you're going right and areas which need improvement.

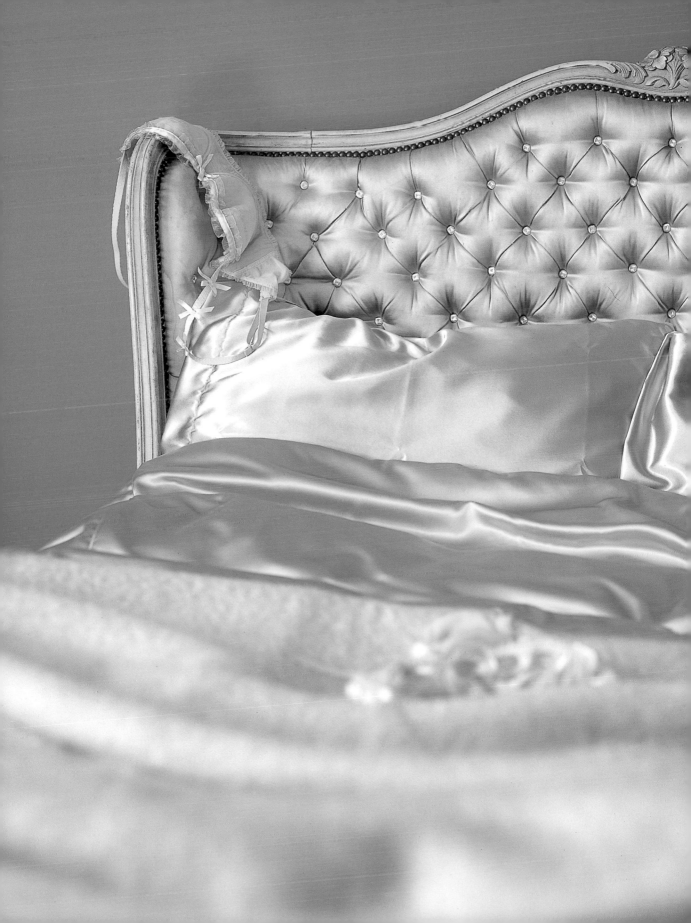

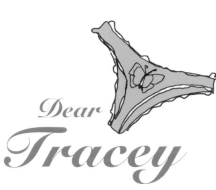

Dear *Tracey*

WHY DON'T WOMEN SUGGEST KINKY THINGS? WHY IS IT LEFT UP TO MEN?

Despite so-called sexual equality, there's still a huge chasm between what men and women are 'supposed' to enjoy. Evidence: I'm talking with a friend of mine, who enthusiastically agrees that it's finally okay for women to sleep with as many people as men do. 'Absolutely! No question!' 'So, if Ellen confessed she'd slept with forty men – which is about how many women you've slept with – you wouldn't mind at all.' He drops his eyes. 'Well, no, that's different. She's my girlfriend,' he mumbles. So there you have it: it's okay for women 'in general' – floating out there somewhere in the universe – to do it, just not anyone men want to get romantically involved with. So when you ask us what we'd really like in bed, we're loath to tell the truth. I know what women's sex fantasies are because I research them for books and it isn't the old 'making love on the beach to a glorious sunset' which tops the list. Women's fantasies are far more ribald, outrageous and kinky. (Just pick up any of Nancy Friday's books.) If you let her know she won't be judged, no matter what she suggests, you might be amazed how far you'll get.

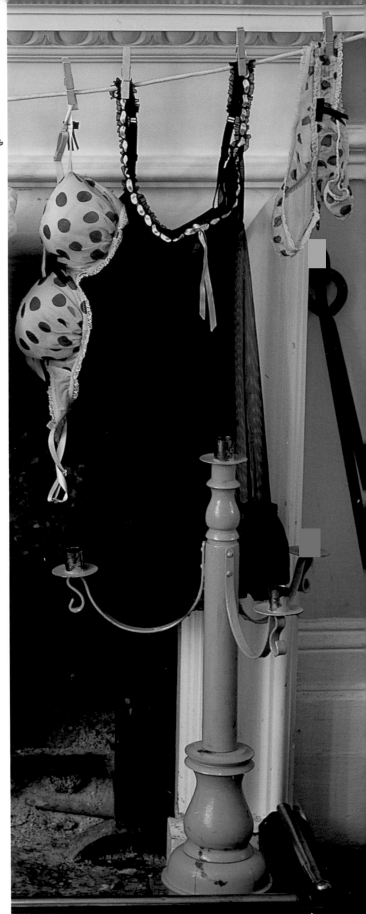

how to tell someone
they're rubbish in bed

AS WELL AS THE TRILLION OTHER QUESTIONS people ask me about this (What do I do if my partner is humiliated/mortified/hates me/shoots me/divorces me/throws themselves in front of a train, etc), the main one people seem to grapple with is how to introduce the topic of 'honey let's fix our sex life' in the first place.

There are several sneaky ways to do this. The first is to use something in the newspaper/magazine you're reading. Point to an article about someone having an affair and then say, 'Honestly! That's the fifty billionth person this week who's cheating on their partner. And I bet it's about sex! (Often it isn't, but that's not important here). Are you happy with our sex life darling? Because I want us both to be completely and utterly satisfied!' They'll mutter something appropriate and that's when you step in with 'Is there anything you'd like me to do in bed that I'm not doing already? There are so many things we could try.' At this stage, they'll still probably think you're after reassurances of fidelity but it's relatively simple to turn it around. Look thoughtful, tap your finger on your chin and say something like, 'Actually, now I think about it, the last time we had sex, I wasn't quite sure whether you were enjoying what I was doing or not ...'

And before you know it, you're (hopefully) chatting about what they'd like more or less of and it's relatively easy from there to guide it to what you'd like more or less of. If prompting the discussion by referring to affairs frightens the life out of you, say you had a dream that the two of you split up and it was truly awful. Hug them and say, 'I'd hate that to happen. Are you happy with our relationship? What about our sex life ...?' And continue as explained before.

Okay, now you've got the gist of it, here are the nitty-gritty details to make it as painless as possible for both of you.

Are you happy with our sex life, darling?

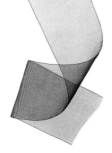

Good things to try

● IF THINGS ARE BAD, DON'T TALK IN THE BEDROOM That's where all the action probably doesn't happen, so it's a no-go zone. Ideally, you'd choose somewhere both of you feel comfortable and share nice 'couple' memories. If you're both 'snuggle up and watch telly' types, talk on the sofa you usually sit on (that's with the telly off, obviously!). If your best time together is when you're both cooking dinner, bring it up while you're pottering about in the kitchen. You can always stop what you're doing to talk. What's important is that the environment feels non-threatening.

● INTRODUCE THE TOPIC IN A LIGHT-HEARTED WAY Saying, 'Sit down, we need to talk,' works for some but terrifies others. I'd suggest not beginning the discussion with, 'We need to talk about our sex life,' or (even worse) 'I'm not happy with our sex life.' (The only time I would suggest this is if your partner is avoiding talking about it and it's a desperate last resort.) The reason why you shouldn't be direct is because people stop listening when they hear something shocking or hurtful. If you say, 'I hate it when you give me oral sex,' they won't hear anything you say after that, even if it's, 'but you are absolutely fantastic at everything else.' They'll be stuck back at 'Ohmigod, she/he thinks I'm crap at oral sex,' for about half an hour, possibly more (days, months, years). It's for this reason you really must …

The reason you shouldn't be direct is because people stop listening when they hear something hurtful

● START WITH THE POSITIVES Saying, 'When you kiss me, I almost throw up,' won't score you sexual brownie points or see an improvement in their kissing technique. Instead, start by complimenting them on what they are getting right (even if it's 'I love the way you look at me when we kiss'). Or try pretending they are already doing what you like. Say, 'I love it when you kiss me really softly,' even if they never have, and it'll ensure that the next time they do kiss you, they'll be more gentle.

● SAY WHAT YOU WANT MORE OF, NOT LESS OF Again, it's all psychological. Asking someone to stop doing something is a negative. Asking them to do more of something is a positive. Instead of, 'When you touch my penis, I can hardly feel it. It's almost like you're scared of it,' say, 'I love it when you touch my penis. Can you do it a bit harder?'

Asking someone to stop doing something is a negative Asking them to do more of something is a positive

● DO UNTO OTHERS Most people do to their partners what they'd like done to them. If you're a sucker for your neck being nibbled, it's likely you'll nibble theirs. Give them the attention you'd like in bed and an astute lover will get the hint: it's rare to do something to someone you don't like yourself. This obviously works in reverse, so pay attention.

● USE BODY LANGUAGE When they do something you like, don't just think, 'At last!'; let them know they've hit the spot. Over exaggerate your response so they can't help but get the message: groan and moan, press yourself closer to them, kiss harder, say 'ummmm'. If you don't like what they're doing, do the opposite. Pull back slightly, twist away and redirect their hand/mouth/bits to where you'd prefer it.

● DON'T REJECT, REDIRECT If he's touching your breast and you don't like it, take his hand and put it somewhere you would like to be touched. Pushing away someone's hand is rude and a turn-off. Lifting it to place it somewhere else, with a sexy, cheeky expression on your face, is a turn-on.

● GIVE AN EXPLANATION Why don't you like what your partner is doing? Is it because it hurts? It's perfectly acceptable to say, 'Ouch! That's hurts!' in a joky way. Generally, men touch women too hard and women touch men too softly. If he/she gets offended, explain it's just a boy/girl thing. Men's skin is thicker and needs a firmer touch, women's skin is thinner and more sensitive, so soft usually works best. If they're very easily offended, word it like this: 'God, that feels delicious (even though it obviously doesn't!) – can you do it a bit harder/softer?' Keep directing till they get it right and then – and this bit's crucial – reward all that hard work with 'Oh God, that's just perfect!' Waxing lyrical about how fabulous they've just made you feel will well and truly soothe any paranoia about having to be directed.

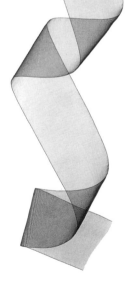

Whatever you do, don't

DON'T TALK IMMEDIATELY AFTER THINGS HAVE GONE HORRIBLY WRONG Erupting into a frenzied, frustrated rant while the bedsprings are still bouncing will guarantee that the problem you've just had has now become a BIG one even if it wasn't before. If sex hasn't gone to plan, acknowledge it lightheartedly, 'Well, we need to work on that. Let's have a chat tomorrow when we're less tired.' Any discussion about sex needs to be treated with tact and sensitivity. You need to think through what you want to say and how you're going to say it – and that's not going to happen if you're in the middle of a red rage.

● **DON'T TALK WHEN YOU'VE JUST HAD A HUGE ROW** Relationship guru John Gottman has done numerous studies on angry couples. These studies all show that people are so flooded with adrenalin when angry, they can't listen effectively or explain their points calmly. Even if the fight was about sex and now seems the perfect time to finally talk about it, wait at least twenty minutes. That's the period of time it takes for the body to return to normal, if you spend it doing some type of calming activity (a walk, making a cup of tea, etc).

Any discussion about sex needs to be treated
with tact, discretion and sensitivity

● **DON'T INITIATE THE DISCUSSION** when the football/their favourite TV show's on/they've got an important work presentation the next day/your three year old's just snuggled up on your lap. Choosing to talk about something as important as this when you're not guaranteed full attention is a waste of time.

● **DON'T BE TOO BOSSY** I know you're rolling your eyes and saying, 'Well, she can hardly talk. She can be a right bossy cow on *The Sex Inspectors*.' But that's different. I'm not that person's partner; I'm someone who they've invited into their home to dispense advice. I have to sound like I know what I'm talking about or else they're not going to trust my advice, are they? You, on the other hand, are intimately involved with the person you're instructing. Your tone should be warm and loving.

Want to have
Great Sex?
Work out what turns you on ...

BEFORE YOU EVEN THINK ABOUT TALKING TO YOUR PARTNER ABOUT WAYS TO MAKE SEX BETTER, YOU NEED A GOOD WORKING KNOWLEDGE OF A PERSON WHO'S CRUCIAL TO YOUR SEXUAL SATISFACTION: YOU! *Unless you know what turns you on and what doesn't,* ANY DISCUSSION ABOUT SEX IS RENDERED POINTLESS BEFORE IT EVEN STARTS. IF YOU'VE GOT A HIGH SEX DRIVE AND LOTS OF GOOD EXPERIENCES WITH SEX, YOU CAN PROBABLY RATTLE OFF A DOZEN THINGS THAT DO IT FOR YOU. *People with a lower sex drive* SOMETIMES AREN'T AS WELL CONNECTED WITH THEIR SEXUAL SELVES. OTHERS STARTED OUT WITH A STRONG, LUSTY INTEREST IN SEX BUT HAVE LOST INTEREST AND ENTHUSIASM ALONG THE WAY AND SIMPLY FORGOTTEN WHAT THEY LIKE AND DON'T. *Whatever situation you're in,* THE FOLLOWING EXERCISES ARE DESIGNED TO HELP YOU BE AS SPECIFIC AS POSSIBLE ABOUT WHAT YOU NEED TO BE HAPPY SEXUALLY. GIVE THEM A WHIRL EVEN IF YOU'RE REASONABLY CONFIDENT – *you may well discover even more about yourself?*

clever communication

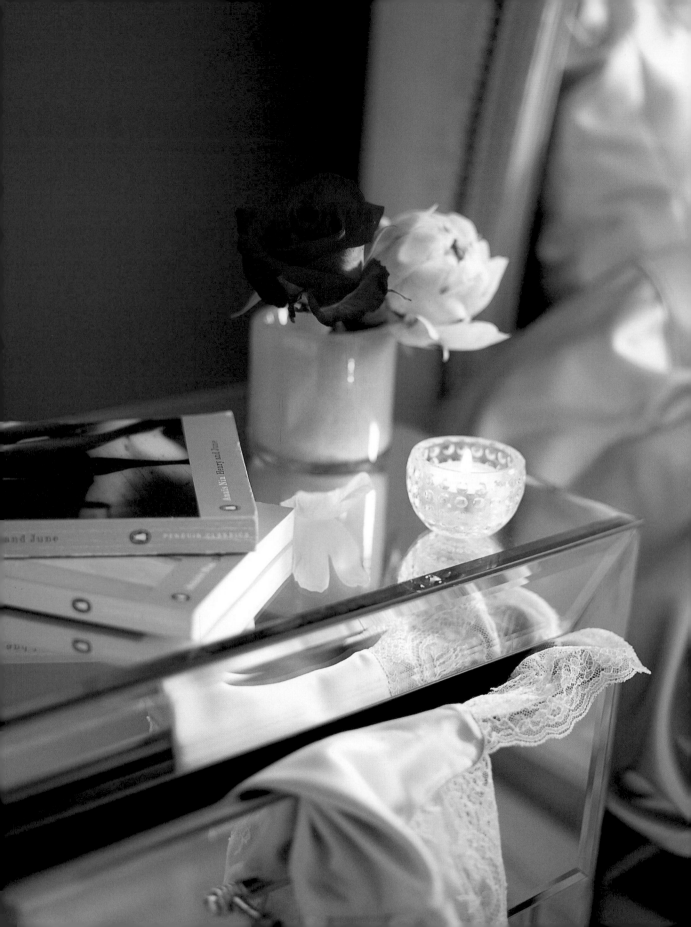

THE AROUSAL CHART

WHY IT WORKS: Our desire levels are fairly predictable. When you're single, abstinence makes any sex feel good because you've gone without it for a while. When you're at the beginning of a relationship, the thrill of new flesh translates to raw lust, which again makes even okay sex feel great. Most of us sail through the initial stage, enthusiastically and merrily shagging away, without too many problems – or too much thought to what we're doing. Just when the novelty starts to wear off, real life (ignored and sulky friends and bosses) kicks back in and sex tends to take a back seat. Early sex is fuelled by passion – a brilliant smokescreen for hiding what the two of you are actually doing to each other. Long-term sex is fuelled by technique, imagination and effort. In other words, the longer you stay together, the more you need to know exactly what turns you on, where/when/how. The more specific you are and the more you each know about your 'triggers' (places or things which never fail to make you aroused), the easier it is to keep your sex life steamy. Once the 'newness' wears off, your libidos both naturally plummet and you have to work at turning yourself and each other on because desire is no longer automatic. This is easier than it sounds. It simply requires knowing yourself inside and out – literally. This exercise helps you do just that: rediscover things you'd forgotten about or discover new things you didn't know you liked.

PROPS YOU'LL NEED: Some sort of pinboard. Pins. Some plain white cards. A private place in your bedroom to hang it but where you'll also see it at least twice daily.

HOW IT WORKS: You're going to make a list of 'sex favourites', write them on the white cards, stick them on the pinboard and update them twice a week for a month (or once a day for seven days if you're particularly motivated/not terribly busy right now/on holidays). I want you to look at the pinboard and really think about what you've written and what you're going to write next. The idea is to focus on sex, to build desire and understand what makes you want to snog your partner senseless when it's been a long, hard day and all you really want to do in bed is sleep. Think about how appealing food is

The thrill of new flesh translates to raw lust, which makes okay sex feel great

All of a sudden you're ravenous

when you walk past a restaurant and you get a delicious waft of your favourite food. Even if you weren't hungry, all of a sudden you're ravenous! Flicking through a foodie magazine, watching seductive chocolate ads, all work to give us an appetite. This does exactly the same thing, except with sex. You're actively stimulating desire rather than expecting it to tap you on the shoulder. Here's a sample of the sort of things you could use as headings for the cards:

WHAT'S MY FAVOURITE PLACE TO HAVE SEX? WHAT'S MY FAVOURITE TIME OF THE DAY TO HAVE SEX? *What's my favourite kissing technique?* WHERE DO I LIKE BEING KISSED MOST? WHAT POSITION/PLACE DO I FIND BEST TO GIVE MY PARTNER ORAL SEX? WHAT POSITION/PLACE/TECHNIQUE DO I LIKE BEST WHEN RECEIVING ORAL SEX? *What's one thing I'd like more of sexually?* WHAT'S ONE THING I COULD LIVE WITHOUT? WHAT'S MY FAVOURITE PART OF FOREPLAY? *What's my favourite part of my body?* WHAT'S MY FAVOURITE PART OF THEIR BODY? WHAT PART OF MY BODY DO I MOST LIKE BEING KISSED/TOUCHED/LICKED? WHAT PART OF THEIR BODY DO I MOST LIKE KISSING/TOUCHING/LICKING? MY FAVOURITE FANTASY IS ... *It turns me on during sex if I'm wearing ...* IT TURNS ME ON DURING SEX IF THEY'RE WEARING ... MY FAVOURITE POSITION FOR INTERCOURSE IS? I LIKE INTERCOURSE MOST WHEN IT'S FAST/SLOW/LASTS FOR (HOW LONG)?

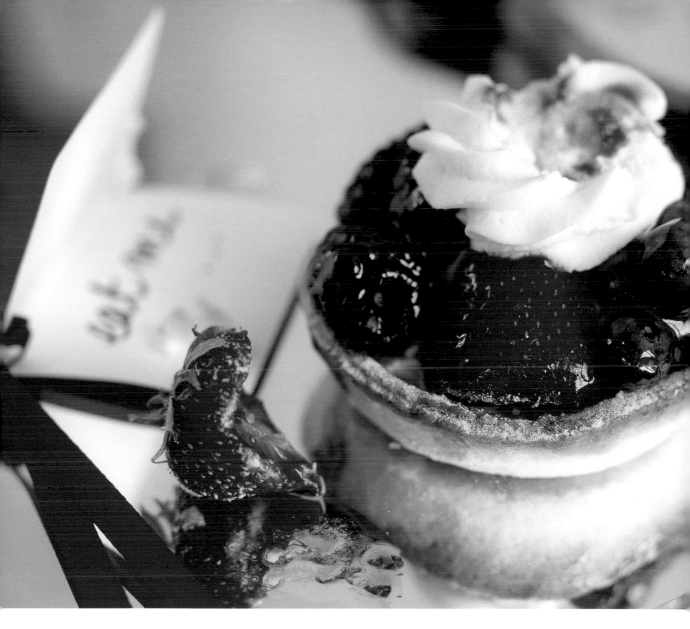

Update the cards regularly but keep the old ones pinned underneath. **WHAT NOW?** This exercise works if you do it solo, then share the results with your partner at the end or if you do it with them, sharing your thoughts as you go along. Just one of you can do it or both of you can do it simultaneously or separately. One word of warning: if you're shy and intend doing the exercise without ever telling your partner what it revealed, you'd better be one hell of a good non-verbal communicator. The point of figuring out what turns you on is so they can help do it!

THE BED PICNIC

WHY IT WORKS: This is a favourite technique of mine because it's both effective and adaptable. Basically, it involves both of you jumping into bed armed with a whole host of goodies, including an armful of sex books. The idea is that you look through the books for ideas on new things you'd like to try, getting you both to talk openly about sex. If you get embarrassed easily or aren't terribly articulate, it's much easier to point to a picture and say, 'I'd like to try that', than it is to say, 'I'd like you to buy a Batman suit and I'll pretend I'm Robin and you come up from behind …'

Props you'll need: Wine, beer, bubbles, fancy cocktails (the more of a 'treat' you make it, the better), exotic food to nibble on (chocolate dipped strawberries, pistachio nuts), food you can feed each other/smear all over (honey, ice-cream, yoghurt). One bedroom and about ten great sex books. It's well worth making the investment and buying them, or pop along to a library and borrow them (just be aware the selection may be a little tame). Make sure you get a selection of topics and authors (Kama Sutra, orgasm focused, hand and oral techniques, fantasy books and good all-rounders like this one) to get a broad range of ideas.

Have a laugh, have a drink, eat some food, snog yourselves stupid, enjoy yourselves

HOW IT WORKS: You can look through the books together or, if you're embarrassed, flick through them separately and simply earmark the pages or put post-it notes on stuff which appeals. When you're finished, swap and then agree on things you'd like to follow through on, making sure they put a sparkle in both your eyes. Once you've done your homework, have some fun. Try some things out there and then, reading out the naughty bits as foreplay. Have a laugh, have a drink, eat some food, snog yourselves stupid, enjoy yourselves!

WHAT NOW? Aim to have a bed picnic at least once every three months. Done well, it should set you up with enough new ideas to keep things nicely varied in between.

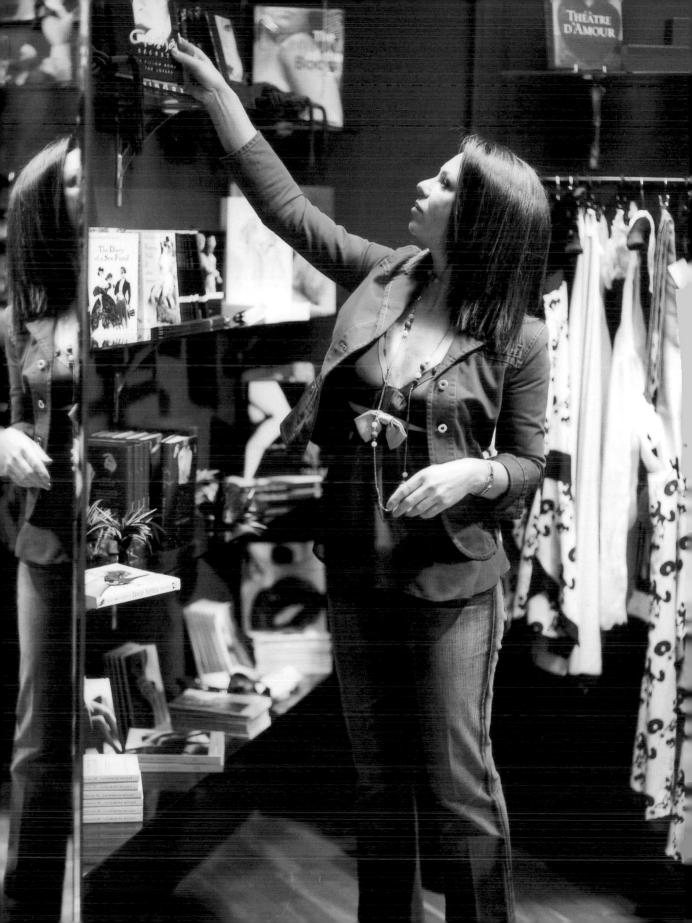

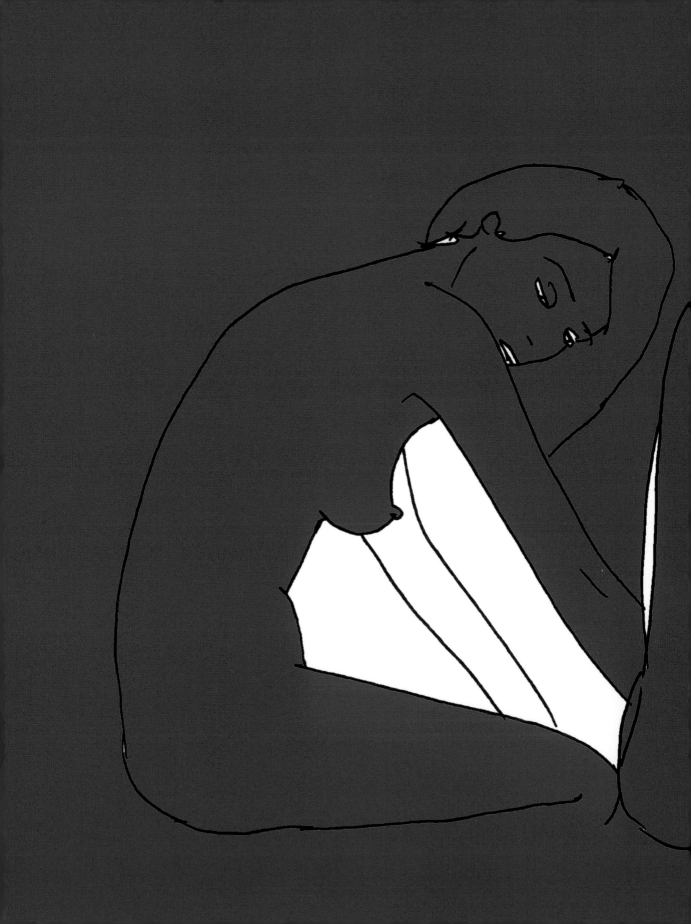

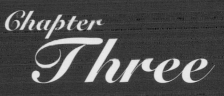

Chapter
Three

problems with parts

Solutions for common sexual problems

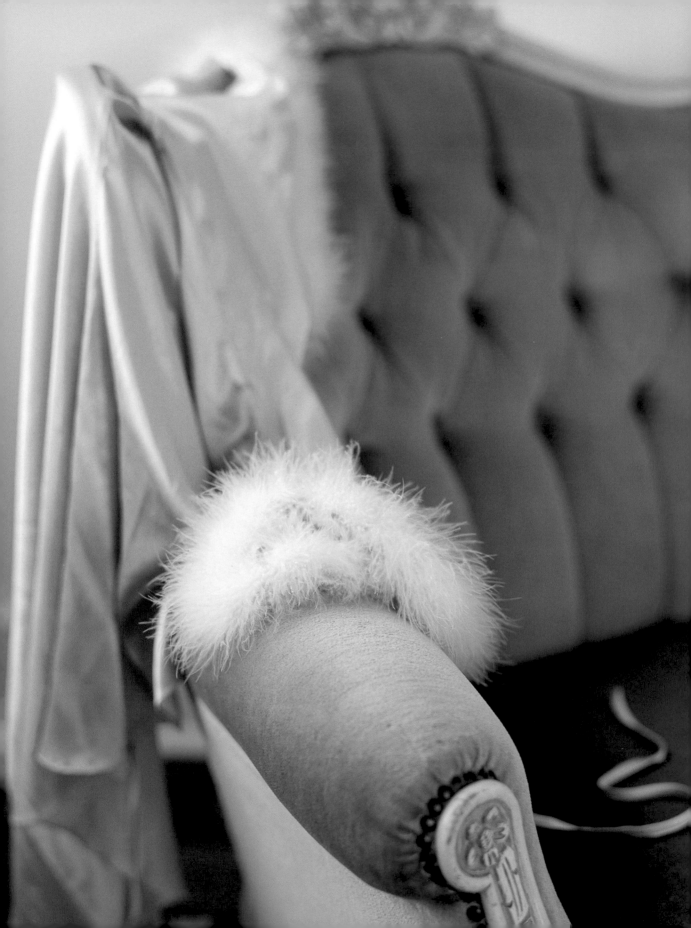

SHAME, CONFUSION, FEAR, ANGER, FRUSTRATION AND SELF-HATRED. These are just a few of the emotions the couples on *The Sex Inspectors* expressed as they struggled with their sexual problems.

'*I feel so humiliated when I can't get an erection that sometimes I just avoid sex.*'

'*I'm so ashamed of my body I can't bear anything but the missionary position.*'

'*I feel like I'm not a real man because I don't want to have sex all the time.*'

'*I don't understand how I can love him so much and want so little sex.*'

I was gutted half the time we were filming. Seeing people so deeply wounded was almost more than I could bear. Couple after couple turned their bedrooms into battlegrounds, declaring occasional truces but no real peace.

Thankfully, we were able to improve the sex lives of all the couples we met on *The Sex Inspectors*. But I couldn't help noticing that some people resolved their sexual problems faster than others. Take Mark and Gary for example. They both had the same problem – premature ejaculation. But one resolved it faster than the other, even though I gave them the same instructions. Why? Because one of them understood a key concept in sexual problem solving: you're weakened by what you're against and strengthened by what you're for.

If you're against premature ejaculation ('I can't stand my girlfriend's look of disappointment when I finish in a minute.'), instead of for staying power ('I want to pleasure my partner until she begs me to stop.') you're in for a long, tough fight. Being against something leaves you hopeless and helpless; being for something leaves you hopeful and optimistic. Concentrating on what you want instead of what you don't want is the fastest way of healing your sexual problems. This principle is all the more important when you understand that the source of most sexual problems is psychological, not medical. They're caused by stress, worry and lack of knowledge,

Concentrating on what you want instead of what you don't want is the fastest way of healing your sexual problems

which lead to harmful interpretations and unhelpful responses.

The people we worked with who got the most out of their experience in *The Sex Inspectors* didn't think their failures were a statement of their self-worth. And neither should you. They didn't fail and say, 'I'm rubbish.' They failed and said, 'Oh, that didn't work. I wonder if this will.'

Free yourself from the idea that you can't be helped. It isn't true. You may be in pain but you don't have to suffer. Your sex life can be infinitely better than it is right now and this chapter will show you how.

Some sexual problems like low libido affect both men and women, but for the most part problems are gender-specific. So let's start with the people who are most likely not to say or do anything about the challenges they face in bed.

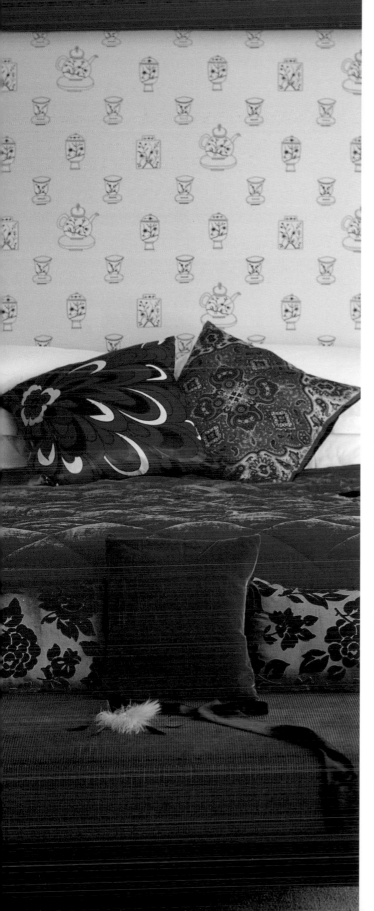

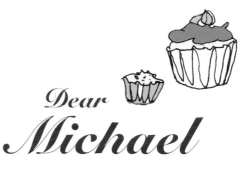

Dear *Michael*

SOMETIMES MY GIRLFRIEND'S VAGINA HAS A 'FISHY' ODOUR, ESPECIALLY AFTER WE HAVE SEX. I KNOW SHE BATHES REGULARLY, SO WHAT CAUSES THIS SMELL AND WHAT CAN BE DONE TO AVOID IT?

Every healthy vagina produces chemicals that keep the area mildly acidic and therefore inhospitable to unhealthy organisms. A 'fishy' odour coming from her vagina might indicate that your girlfriend has an infection called bacterial vaginosis. Doctors don't concur on one single cause for BV: it can occur when other, less friendly bacteria are introduced through outside sources like douching, wiping from back to front after a bowel movement (which carries germs from the anus to the vagina), or even getting used to a new penis. Oh, oh. Oops, never mind! A doctor can treat BV with pills or cream. BV is relatively common; some estimates say that as many as sixty-four per cent of women have the infection at any one time.

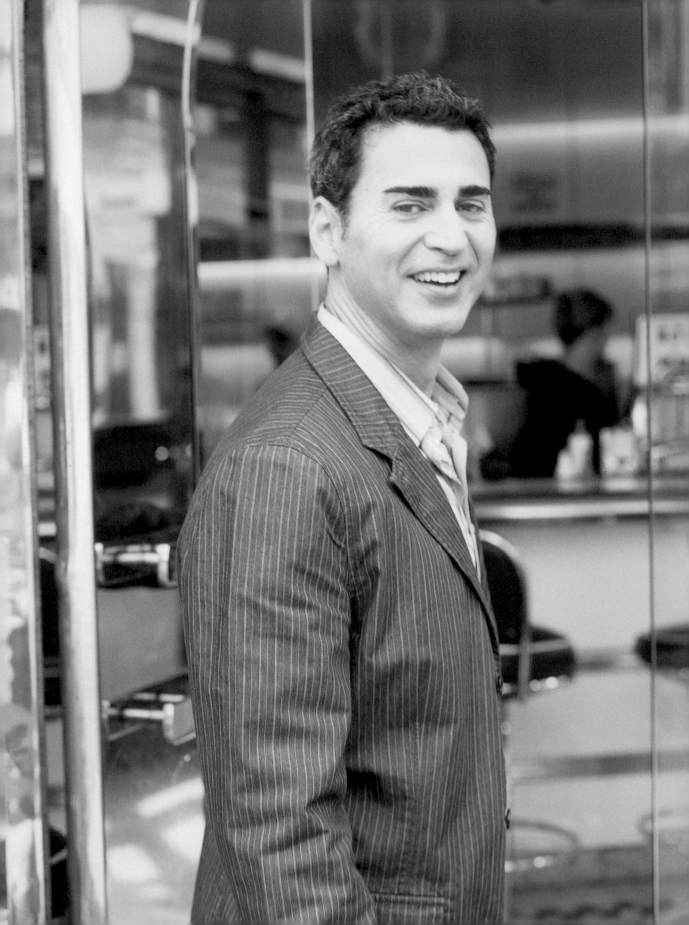

For Him

THEY SAY THAT IF TYRES OR TESTICLES are involved, there'll be trouble. And the trouble with men can be divided into three parts: getting it up, getting it out and getting it on (impotence, ejaculation and technique).

PREMATURE EJACULATION

Premature ejaculation is the most common sexual dysfunction in men under forty. About thirty per cent of men complain about it. Men have subconsciously trained themselves into ejaculating prematurely. As boys we learned to masturbate quickly. After all, how long can you stay in the bathroom with your mum banging on the door screaming, 'WHAT ARE YOU DOING IN THERE??!!!' But before you label yourself a Three-Stroke Bloke, know that the average session of intercourse lasts about five minutes. So even if your partner uses your sessions as an egg timer you're halfway to average. One condom manufacturer said they only need to test their product for fifty thrusts. Doesn't say much for male stamina, does it? Still, the question remains: how quick is too quick? How do you define premature ejaculation? Easy. It's the inability to consciously control or choose when to climax. Mark, one of the contributors on *The Sex Inspectors*, was a premature ejaculator. He tried to last longer the way most guys do: by counting to 100, or picturing things that turned him off – like dead cats, his bank statements, that sort of thing. He couldn't have picked a worse strategy. The problem wasn't that he was paying too much attention to his body; it was that he wasn't paying enough.

I helped Mark with the first step in overcoming premature ejaculation: identifying and avoiding the point of 'ejaculatory inevitability'. Or, in plain English, 'the point of no return'.

The average session of intercourse lasts about 5 minutes

Like all premature ejaculators, Mark was basically skipping the 'plateau' stage, where all the action is (See Chapter One). He wasn't aware of the subtle cues leading to his orgasms. By using the Stop/Start/Change method Mark went from a two-pump chump to a long-time champ. If it worked for him it'll work for you. Here's how to do it:

STOP/START ALONE. When you're alone, masturbate until you get close to the 'point of no return', then STOP. Do nothing but focus on the sensation of your penis. The urge to orgasm will subside within three minutes. Start masturbating again. Do this over and over and you'll find you'll last longer and longer. When you've got that down, go to step two.

PACE ALONE. Now masturbate until you get close to coming and instead of stopping, slow down. CHANGE. Change the speed of your stroke, the pressure you put on it and the site of your grip. Take your hand away from the head where there's more sensation to the shaft where there's less.

STOP/START TOGETHER. Have your partner masturbate you until you get close to ejaculatory inevitability then have her STOP. Basically, follow step one, only your partner's doing the work and you're doing the refereeing.

PACE TOGETHER. Now have your partner masturbate you until you get close to coming and instead of stopping, CHANGE. Basically, follow step two.

INTERCOURSE ON YOUR BACK. Lie flat on your back with your partner sitting on top. Do NOT use the missionary position because it uses your muscles differently and it's harder to get relaxed. Insert your erect penis into her. Don't move. Get acclimatized for as long as it takes. Now use the stop/start/change method. You move up and down. Getting close? Stop. Wait a few minutes. Now have her move up and down. Close? Change.

GRADUATING TO THE MISSIONARY POSITION. Enter her when you're on top. Start moving. S-l-o-w-l-y. Keep using the Stop/Start/Change method throughout.

Quickie Tip

AS YOU GET CLOSER TO ORGASM YOUR TESTICLES MOVE UP TOWARDS YOUR BODY. BY PULLING THEM DOWN YOU CAN DELAY ORGASM. IF YOU FEEL YOURSELF GETTING CLOSE, GET YOUR PARTNER TO GRAB YOUR SCROTUM JUST ABOVE THE TESTICLES AND TUG GENTLY

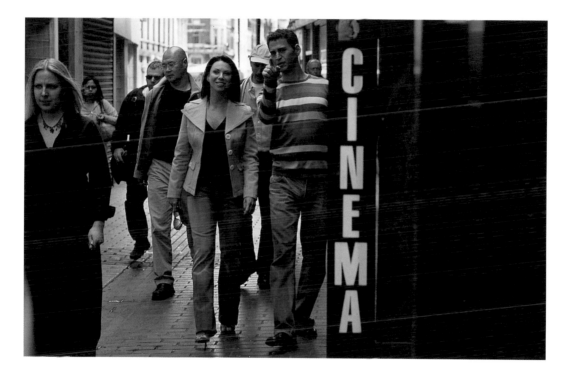

DELAY AWAY Never use creams or ointments that claim they'll help you last longer. They don't work and you'll end up rubbing it off on your partner, causing her a loss of sensation. On top of that, she may be allergic to its active ingredient, benzocaine . Think she'll forgive you for taking her to the emergency room when all she wanted was to be taken? France doesn't grow enough roses to get you out of that one.

IMPOTENCE

Impotence is the most common problem affecting men over forty. Up to a third of erectile dysfunction is physical, but 90 per cent of problems are treatable. If you're having problems, then get it checked out with your doctor. Here are the major medical reasons for impotence and possible solutions:

● **DISEASES** Anything that impedes blood flow to the penis is going to give it a flat tyre. That includes obesity, diabetes, atherosclerosis (hardening of the arteries), high blood pressure and nervous system diseases like multiple sclerosis.

SOLUTION Eat healthily, exercise regularly, stop smoking (it constricts blood vessels leading to the penis), and take appropriate medication.

● **PHYSICAL TRAUMA** Spinal cord injuries, for example. Or getting kicked in the groin (accidentally in a football game, or purposefully by an ex-girlfriend).

SOLUTION Take up a new sport, get a court order against your ex-girlfriend, or take drugs like papaverine and phentolamine, which you inject into your penis with a hypodermic needle. It isn't the most romantic thing in the

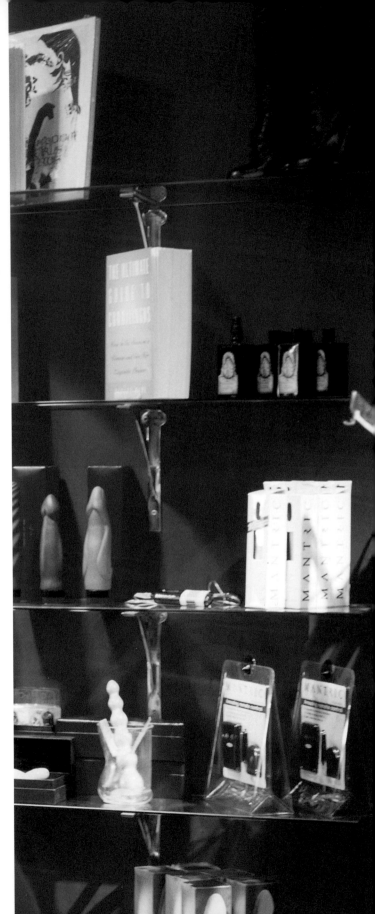

world, but it works. You can also get surgical implants that give you an erection by pumping saline water into your penis.

● MEDICATIONS Over 200 commonly prescribed drugs cause or contribute to impotence, including drugs for high blood pressure, heart medications, antidepressants, tranquillizers and sedatives. Even some over-the-counter medications can make your putter sputter.

SOLUTION Switch medications. For instance, some anti-depressants cause fewer sexual side effects than others. Or add medications that counteract the side effects of your must-have pills. If none of that works, there's also Alprostadil, a pellet you insert into the opening of your penis and push into the urethra. If you think that's too romantic for words then try the vacuum pump. You stick your penis into a plastic cylinder and prime the pump. That creates a vacuum, which pulls blood into the penis. Wrap an elastic band around the base of your penis and you're good to go.

Around forty, the average man's testosterone level starts to drop by fifteen per cent each decade

● DRUGS AND ALCOHOL They're great at lowering inhibitions but they can make sex harder than shooting pool with a rope. Chronic use of drugs and alcohol can affect parts of the vascular and nervous systems associated with erections.

SOLUTION Straight from the Department of Duh: Stop Using Them. I know, you work hard during the week and you want to get off your face on the weekend. Fine. You just won't get on hers. If you give a urine sample and a cocktail olive comes out it's time to quit altogether. If not, at least cut back.

● PHYSIOLOGICAL CHANGES Around forty, the average man's testosterone level starts to drop by fifteen per cent each decade. If that doesn't give you vertigo I don't know what will. Since testosterone is the fuel that makes the libido take off, make sure you have enough of it.

SOLUTION Get your testosterone levels checked. If they're low you've got three choices: pill, patch or shot. They work but beware: adding testosterone tends to 'teach' your body to make less testosterone on its own, creating a cycle of depletion hard to overcome. Also, if you show even a hint of prostate cancer (the biggest cancer killer in men) taking testosterone is like spraying Miracle Grow on it. Ask your doctor what's right for you.

Not every case of erectile dysfunction is caused by a physical condition. There are also psychological factors.

● EMOTIONAL TRAUMA Forced sex, incest or harassment can severely impact sexual performance. So can other traumas like growing up in a harshly negative upbringing where you were taught that sex was dirty or an evil sin.

SOLUTION Therapy. By talking things out, healing painful memories and learning new ways of thinking and behaving, you'll discover new springs in your mattress.

● STRESS Anything that causes high anxiety, for example work, divorce, exams or financial worries.

SOLUTION Meditate, do yoga, fire your boss, try progressive muscle relaxation exercises, make time to reflect, relax and rejuvenate. Try hypnosis, which studies have shown can reduce pain and anxiety. Know that 'situational impotence' is temporary and happens to everyone. Once the stressor is removed, your penis will move.

Once the stress is removed, your penis will move

How do you know if you need a doctor?

TAKE A TEST: IF YOU CAN MASTURBATE OR GET A DAYTIME OR NOCTURNAL ERECTION, THEN YOU DON'T NEED A DOCTOR. IF YOU CAN'T GET AN ERECTION AT ALL UNDER ANY CIRCUMSTANCES, THEN THERE'S PROBABLY SOMETHING WRONG WITH YOUR HYDRAULICS, SO PICK UP THE PHONE AND MAKE AN APPOINTMENT.

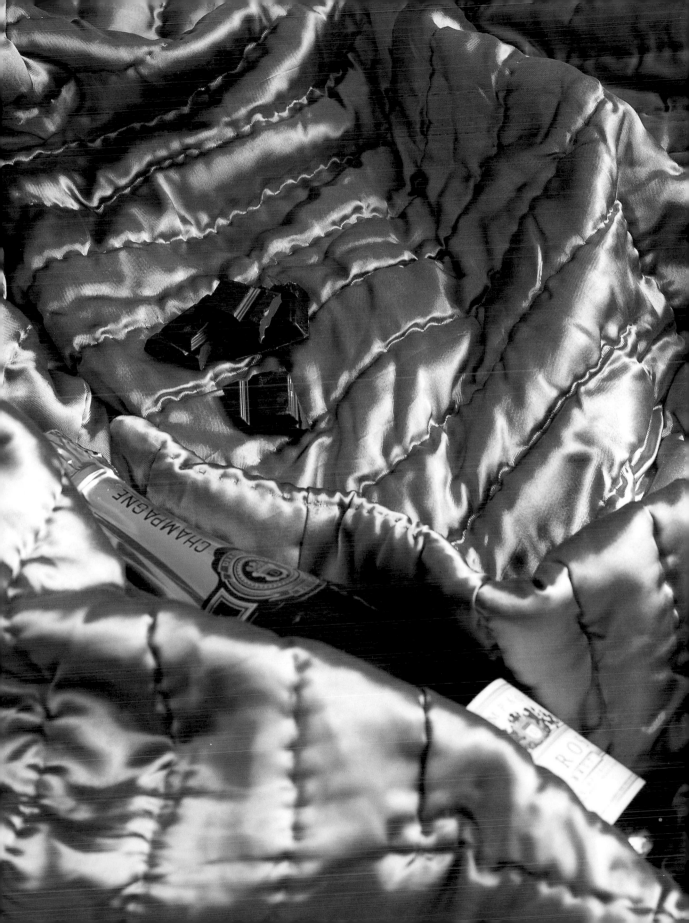

PUTTING IMPOTENCE ON THE RUN

No emotional issues? No medical issues? Can't take erectile dysfunction drugs because you have high blood pressure? Then run like hell. Studies show that active men have a thirty per cent lower risk of impotence than men who sit on their arses eating crisps. The fitter the man, the stronger the erection. Any aerobic activity (running, football, biking) produces the most benefit.

Quickie questions

● SOMETIMES, RIGHT BEFORE I EJACULATE I GET CRAMPS IN MY LEGS Cramps during sex aren't unusual. They're caused by spending too much time in one position. Change positions often, or don't stay in them for very long. Also, are you drinking enough water? Dehydration is one of the most common causes of cramps.

● WHY DO I SOMETIMES HAVE BLOOD IN MY SEMEN? 'Haematospermia', which is blood in the ejaculate, should be checked out immediately, but is more often a scare than a problem. In half the cases there's no known cause for it. If it happens regularly it might be a prostate infection, easily treated with antibiotics.

● I HAD AN ORGASM BUT NOTHING CAME OUT! WHERE DID IT GO? You probably had a temporary 'retrograde ejaculation'. Meaning, instead of the semen being forced out of the urethra it got forced into the bladder. During normal orgasms a tiny muscle at the entrance of the bladder shuts off, but in retrograde ejaculations, that tiny muscle doesn't shut properly, allowing all or part of the semen to travel backwards into the bladder. If it's only happened once I wouldn't worry about it. If it happens more frequently see your doctor.

Sex, Drugs and Rock & Roll

All three erectile dysfunction drugs in the market today operate the same way. They block an enzyme called PDE-5, a chemical that shoos away erections. There's more PDE-5 in the penis than anywhere else in the body and that's why the drugs have such specific effects down there. ED drugs like Viagra don't increase your libido. They improve blood flow to the penis when you get aroused. No arousal, no erection.

STIFFEN YOUR RESOLVE

Should you take erectile dysfunction drugs? Not if you have a heart or blood pressure condition. If you want the thrill of your heart rate dropping to dangerous levels, check your credit card balance instead. There are three erectile dysfunction drugs on the market: **Viagra, Levitra** and **Cialis** (pronounced 'See-Alice'). Each has their upsides and downsides:

Cialis

BENEFITS Can last up to forty-eight hours (the French call it 'Le weekend'), giving you something the others can't – spontaneity. Unlike Viagra, it's as effective on an empty stomach as a full one.
DRAWBACKS The slowest acting of the three, it takes about an hour to get an erection. It can also give you a general achy feeling, especially around the back.

Levitra

BENEFITS Quick erections. You won't have to drum your fingers on the table for more than thirty minutes before you can lay hands upon the wonderment.
DRAWBACKS Can give some men a bluish tint to their vision.

Viagra

BENEFITS Has the longest track record of effectiveness and safety.
DRAWBACKS Food significantly diminishes its effectiveness, so wait three hours after a meal before taking a dose. Also gives vision a bluish tint and sometimes gives headaches.

For her

STUDIES SHOW THAT WOMEN ARE FAR MORE LIKELY than men to suffer from low libido and other sexual dysfunctions. That's because your reproductive system is far more complex. Experts cite four areas that women tend to have the most problems in: desire, arousal, orgasms and vaginal pain.

Adding to the difficulties is the fact that when women suffering with sexual dysfunctions see their physicians they are either too embarrassed to talk about it, feel it's too unimportant to bring up or are convinced that treatments don't exist.

Nothing could be further from the truth. It is not too embarrassing, it is important, and there are treatments available. The next time you're at the doctor's I want you to say, 'I'm having a problem with something I'm a little embarrassed to bring up but it's important to me, so I need you to take the time to listen and advise me on the best treatment options.'

I AM WOMAN, HEAR ME SNORE

The most common problem women face in bed is that they would rather sleep in it than make love in it. This problem comes in two versions: 'Hypoactive Sexual Desire Disorder' and 'Sexual Arousal Disorder'. Not only do these terms sound almost exactly alike, they're so clinical I'm reaching for a white lab coat and I don't even own one! So if you don't mind, I'm going to re-label them **'Low Libido'** and **'Low Sensation'**.

● **'Low Libido'** means you don't want it, you don't think about it, you don't fantasize about it, you're not receptive to it. You'd rather curl up with a good book than a good bloke.

● **'Low Sensation'**, on the other hand, means you want it, but your

The most common problem women face in bed is that they would rather sleep in it than make love in it

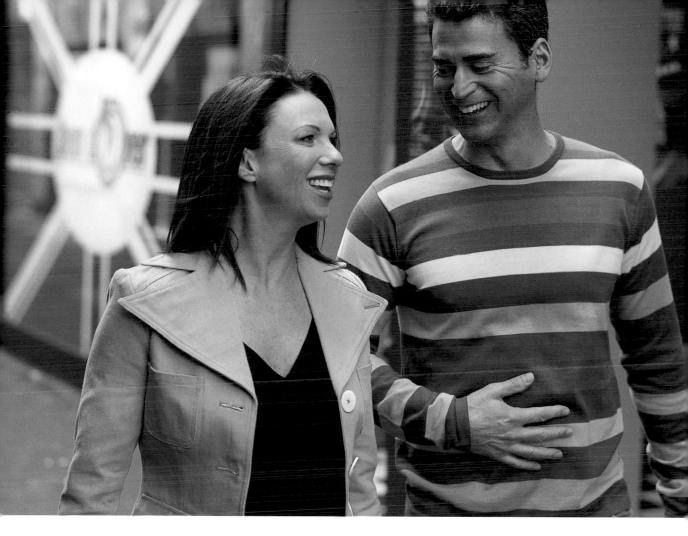

body doesn't. It's a classic case of 'the spirit is willing but the flesh is weak.' And there are very real reasons why it's weak – a measurable lack of lubrication, decreased nipple sensitivity and reduced clitoral and labial sensation. Often women suffering from Low Sensation remember how good sex can be – but they just don't respond to it as they once did.

For decades, 'experts' (usually men) accused women of inventing their own problems, claiming it was 'all in their heads', or attaching lovely labels like 'frigid'. How very helpful. And how very wrong. Today, we know it's not 'all in your head'. There are substantiated physiological reasons why you prefer turning the page than doing the twist. Before we get into what they are and what you can do about it, see Tracey's chapter on low libido for some highly imaginative and effective ways to kick-start your libido without medical treatment.

THE LOW-DOWN ON LOW LIBIDO & LOW SENSATION

Though low libido is clearly linked to psychological or emotional causes, including stress, fatigue and depression, there are often underlying physical causes. The most common culprits:

● PELVIC SURGERY (including hysterectomy) or trauma. Either can restrict blood flow to the sexual nerves, resulting in a loss of sensation.

● HIGH BLOOD PRESSURE, UNCONTROLLED DIABETES, CORONARY HEART DISEASE, SMOKING OR HIGH CHOLESTEROL – all of which result in either constriction or blockage of blood flow to the sexual regions. A healthy blood flow prompts the swelling, engorgement and lubrication necessary for sexual pleasure.

● HORMONAL CHANGES including menopause or having a baby.

● UNDERACTIVE THYROID

● ENDOMETRIOSIS and FIBROIDS

● MEDICATION Some antidepressants, blood pressure medications, anticonvulsants, anticancer drugs and even birth control pills can cause a physical reduction in either sexual arousal or responsiveness.

WHAT YOU CAN DO

There are now many more health professionals going into the field of sexual medicine and psychotherapy, and so there has never been a better time to ask for help. Initially, it's important that your medical, sexual and social history is taken. You may also need tests to check for diabetes, hypertension or blood pressure and for hormone levels, blood pressure. You could also consider asking your doctor for the following tests:

● VAGINAL BLOOD FLOW You can find out the level of blood flow and temperature through a light-reflecting, tampon-shaped device inserted into the vagina.

● VAGINAL PH TESTING This is a routine test gynaecologists and urologists use to detect bacteria-causing vaginitis. Since decreasing hormone levels and diminished vaginal lubrication affect pH balance, you can tell if hormonal imbalances are a contributing factor.

Once your doctor gets the information, he or she can decide on a course of treatment. It's

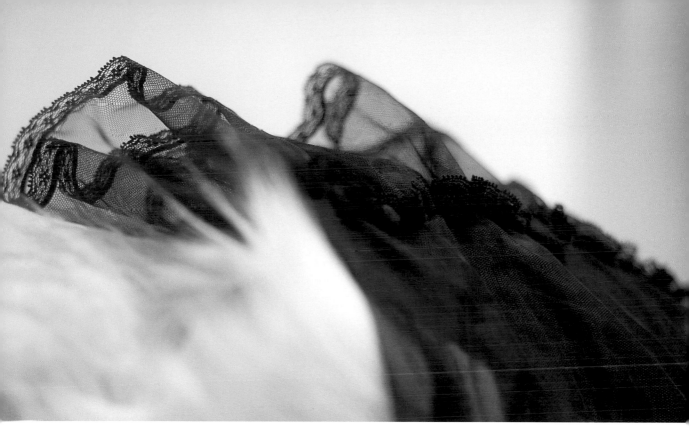

usually some combination of sex therapy, drugs, hormone replacement and sexual enhancing devices. Here's a breakdown of your choices:

● **HORMONE REPLACEMENT THERAPY** Oestrogen, testosterone and other hormones are measured and then balanced. Some women see vast improvements; others see none. There are risky side effects associated with this controversial option so consult carefully with your doctor.

● **VIAGRA** Yes, the little blue pill that makes men's penises stand up and salute can also make your clitoris sit up and beg. Though studies are inconclusive, there are women who've seen their libidos come to life with Viagra, especially if they're on anti-depressants.

● **SEX THERAPY** Your GP or local family planning clinic can tell you where to find your nearest NHS psychosexual service. Sex therapy can help you to explore your feelings about sex and learn more about your body. If you can attend with your partner then all the better, as you will be provided with the perfect supportive atmosphere in which to be open and honest about your issues, whether physical or emotional, or a combination of both.

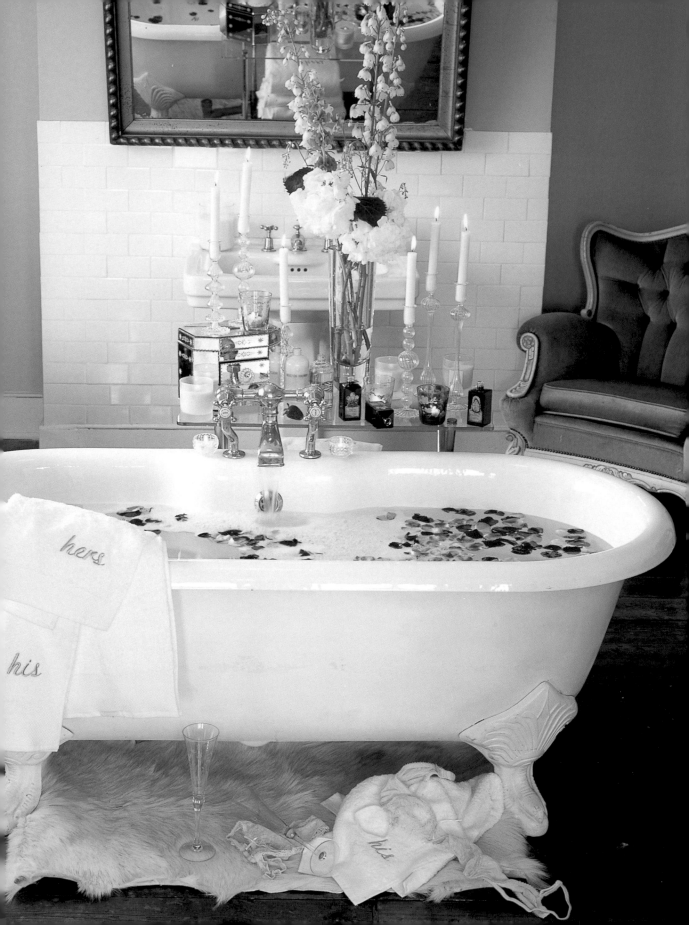

Squeeze until you Wheeze

EXERCISING YOUR VAGINAL MUSCLES WILL IMPROVE YOUR CHANCES OF WANTING SEX AND BEING ABLE TO ORGASM. DO THE KEGEL EXERCISES COVERED IN CHAPTER ONE. THEY'LL IMPROVE BLOOD FLOW TO THE GENITALS.

PAIN WITH INTERCOURSE

Genital pain from intercourse often results from medical problems such as vaginal infections, inflammations or thinning membranes during menopause. Some women even experience a disorder called vaginismus, involuntary muscle spasms in the first third of the vagina. The result is your body hangs a blinking 'no entry' sign on itself. Here's what to do:

● **CONSULT YOUR DOCTOR** Infections and inflammations can be treated. You can also manage menopause symptoms in both traditional and alternative ways.

● **TRY DILATORS** In conjunction with the Kegel exercises, vaginal dilators can help overcome the PC spasm reflex. Dilators come in sets of varying sizes. Start with the smallest and work up to penis size – as you consciously squeeze and relax the PC muscles try inserting the dilator. Gradually you will be able to override the involuntary contractions which previously closed the entrance to the vagina.

● **LOAD UP THE LUBE** Buy it by the barrel. Like good sex, too much is never enough.

GADGET-FREE ALTERNATIVES

● **EXERCISE** The best way to improve blood flow and circulation is to move your body. Go for long walks. Exercise until your face flushes – you just might find other parts flushing too.

● **GET IN HOT WATER** Heat promotes blood circulation. Soak in a hot bath. Not only is it a sensual treat, you may find the relaxation helpful.

● **GIVE UP FOR A WHILE** Swear off penetrative sex for a bit. If the pain is a conditioned response to painful sexual encounters in the past, you may need to retrain your body from its 'flight or fight' response. It's a vicious cycle but a sensitive counsellor can help.

● **GO NATURAL** Talk to your chemist about natural alternatives to improving blood flow. Some people swear by non-prescription solutions containing an amino acid called L-Arginine.

A CRYING SHAME

Experts may not recognize it as an official sexual disorder but after working with couples on *The Sex Inspectors* I'm convinced that the most challenging problem women face in bed is the mirror. Every woman I talked to said the way she felt about her body negatively affected the quality of her sex life. Sarah, for example, was so ashamed of the weight she had gained that she would only have sex in the missionary position. That way her boyfriend couldn't get a full view of her body. The fact that he adored her body made no difference to Sarah.

Every woman in *The Sex Inspectors* had a little Sarah in them. And I bet you do, too. Body shame is so pervasive it leaves almost no woman untouched. When Kinsey worked on his famous study he found that women felt more embarrassed when he asked them about their weight than when he asked them about their masturbation practices or if they had lesbian experiences. And that was in 1953! Women are taught from an early age that their self-worth is largely

It's impossible to have a successful orgasm when you're holding in your stomach

dependent on how they look. The evidence is everywhere. The media assault us with one and only one ideal of feminine beauty – tall, slim women with big chests. 'Stick bugs with breasts', as Bridget Jones put it so memorably in the first movie.

Have you noticed that only great-looking women have sex on the telly? The underlying message is clear: you're not allowed to have an orgasm unless you weigh under 120 pounds. Another supporting fact: in employment, there are only two jobs where women earn more than men: modelling and prostitution.

I'm here to tell you, it's impossible to have a successful orgasm when you're holding your stomach in. It's time to reclaim your right to hot sex even though you don't fit the ideal of a 'stick bug with breasts'.

What you can do ...

● FOCUS AND PAMPER Pick the things you like about your body and pamper them. Is your hair shiny? Buy the best shampoos and conditioners. Are your feet pretty? Get regular pedicures. If you start being grateful for what you like you'll be more forgiving of what you don't.

● FANTASIZE He may not be fantasizing that you're Pamela Anderson in bed, but you can! Use the power of your imagination to ease you into better sex.

● FOCUS ON YOUR PARTNER You can't replace 'A' with 'not A'. You've got to replace it with 'B'. You can't 'not think' about your body. But you can think about another one – his.

● FOCUS ON SENSATIONS, NOT EMOTIONS When you're having sex, go on high alert for physical sensations, not emotional judgments. If you don't like your thighs, fine. But what does the satin sheet underneath them feel like? Don't like your breasts? That's okay. What do they feel like when they're being kissed in just the right way? By focusing your attention on physical sensations you can sidestep your inner critic and sink into the sensuality of your body.

● SHAKE THE BED UP Move around, be more active when you're making love. Why? Because then you're not solely an object to look at but a vehicle for pleasure. It takes your mind away from how you're looking to what you're doing.

What your partner can do ...

● DON'T LOOK THROUGH A *PLAYBOY* AND THEN HIT ON YOUR PARTNER She'll know you were drooling on the kind of 'perfection' she can't live up to. She'll either think another woman made you horny or that you're going to make love to her while thinking about the Playboy Bunny.

● DON'T BUY HER CLOTHES THAT'LL MAKE HER FEEL SELF-CONSCIOUS Skip the thongs and go for something sheer that gives coverage and yet has a naked or semi-naked effect.

● BE SPECIFIC IN YOUR COMPLIMENTS Saying, 'I love you' is fine. Saying, 'It's hard to concentrate at work because I daydream about your legs,' is finer.

the body map

WHY IT WORKS: People often joke and say it's a shame their partners didn't come with an instruction manual. Well, you're about to create one. This exercise will leave you with a map of how and where you like to be touched. After you've done it, you swap with your partner and - voilà! - you've both got an instant instruction guide.

Men, who tend to be mostly visual, respond well to this exercise because they can see what's expected of them sexually. Your needs and wants are clearly spelled out because you're literally charting a map of how your partner can pleasure you. Some people stick the map on the ceiling or walls of their bedroom until they know it off by heart. Others look at it carefully, then chuck it in a cupboard (or the bin, if you're a quick learner). We used The Body Map on Nicky and Andrew, a couple from Brighton who had mismatched libidos. It worked a treat! It's not a 'heavy' exercise and feels more like a game, so it's fun and non-threatening to do. But the secrets it reveals - what your partner really enjoys, as opposed to what you think they enjoy - are enormously helpful.

I always like my nipples to be kissed and licked. Sometimes I also like you to bite them. Mostly I like soft strokes with your fingers, but on lusty days, I like it if you even pinch slightly. The only way to know what I'm in the mood for is to ask.

PROPS YOU WILL NEED: A really large piece of cardboard (you may have to order it from an art shop, or stick smaller sheets together). **Permanent markers or felt-tip pens**: two sets, in black, green, red and blue (or other distinctly different colours).

HOW IT WORKS: Strip NAKED or at least down to your *underwear* and get your partner to draw around you with the black pen, so you end up with an OUTLINE OF YOUR BODY. It doesn't matter if it looks all wobbly and weird, but *life-size* is easier to relate to. Now I want you to go to different places for an hour or so, armed with your pens. The reason you shouldn't do it together is because it's too TEMPTING to look at what your partner is doing, rather than focus on yourself. Now use the red pen to colour in places on your BODY where you don't like being *touched,* no matter what. Red equals NO-GO ZONES, and hopefully there won't be too many of those. Use the blue pen to colour in areas which are MOOD DEPENDENT - places which feel good at times but not at others - and also places you're sort of LUKEWARM about. Use the green pen on places where you love being touched. Green effectively means *Go for it!* Now, go back to all the places you've coloured blue and green, CIRCLE SPECIFIC AREAS, draw an arrow and use the black pen to write down what you'd like done to that particular area. Lots of detail, please. When you're completely SATISFIED you've covered the main areas, meet up and *swap maps.*

WHAT NOW? It's really important not to get all huffy if your perception of your partner's likes and dislikes doesn't match their map. In fact, prepare to be puzzled, as Nicky was. I don't know one couple who have done this exercise without learning something from it. Remember, it could be the first time your partner has really concentrated on what they like or don't like, rather than just lying back and receiving whatever is given. They might be amazed at what they've written too. True, it is a bit annoying to find out that all the effort you put into playing with a particular body part was pointless, given they'd prefer you to give it a big swerve. But that's the point! It's a good thing to discover new sexual information about each other. A very good thing, because once you both start touching the right places in the right way, your sex life will dramatically improve.

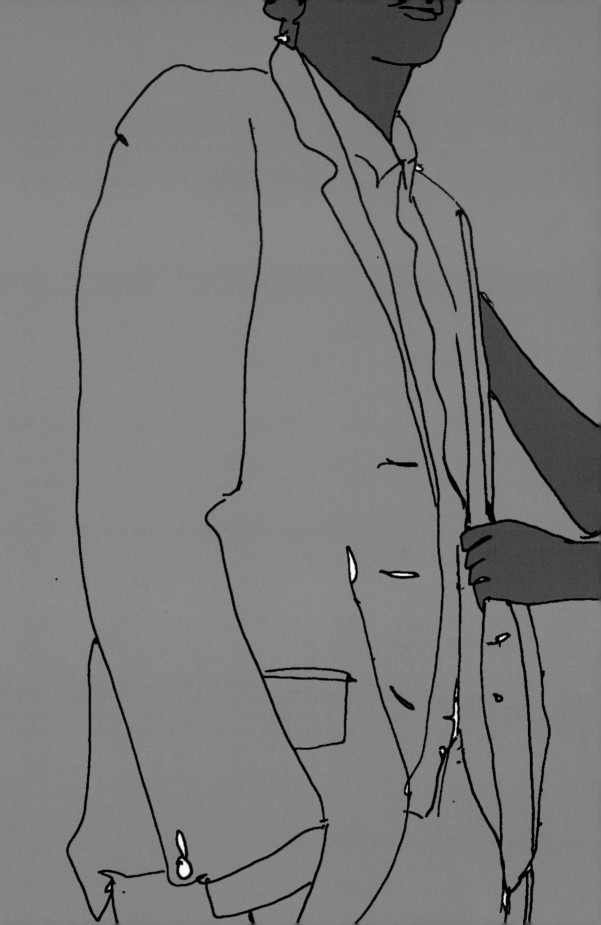

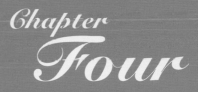

mismatched libidos

Ways to fix a sex-starved marriage and cope with desire doldrums

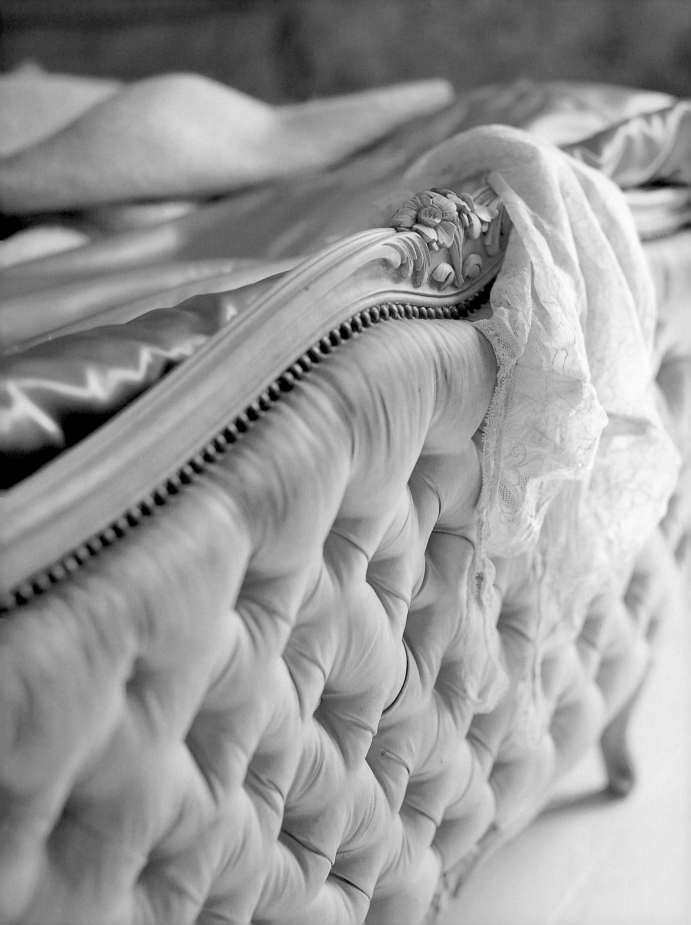

DATING AGENCIES GET IT HORRIBLY WRONG. Forget trying to match people up based on age and a passion for metal detecting. Their success rate would soar if instead they asked one simple question: 'How much do you love sex?' The list of potential hook-ups would then neatly and tidily divide into their relevant groups and they'd know exactly who to match up with whom!

In an ideal world, all high sex drive people would go out with high sex drive people and all low desire people would do likewise. Believe me, your sex lives would be a lot simpler if you did. Studies suggest one in three marriages in Britain and the US struggle with problems associated with mismatched desire – I'd put that figure a lot higher. I mean, it's bound to cause problems if you put someone who'd happily trade a lifetime of telly for one gobsmackingly great sex session, with someone who'd find it hard to feign enthusiasm if Brad Pitt or Angelina Jolie (or both) knocked on the front door, naked, and fell immediately to their knees.

Why, then, do we insist on matching up with people who don't feel about sex the same way we do? Well, one reason is relationships and love aren't based entirely on sex. We fall in love and decide to settle down for lots of reasons, not just sexual compatibility. The other reason is it's really hard to tell in the beginning what sort of sex drive your partner has. Our libido is strongly influenced by hormones and other substances which tend to go bonkers during that heady, hedonistic beginning bit. During infatuation, the body releases high levels of PEA (phenylethylamine) and dopamine, and even people who usually couldn't care less experience a sensational surge in desire. This means someone with quite a low sex drive acts and feels like a person with a high libido (How wonderful! I'm different with this person!). The high sex drive person – who tends to register a consistently high level of testosterone (the primary sex hormone regulating desire in both men and women) is thrilled ('Brilliant! Here's someone who adores sex as much as I do!') Sadly, both have been misled by nature. The hormone boosts don't last and (usually within a few months or at best 18 months), return to their true levels. It's then abundantly clear if you are at opposite extremes.

Happily, there's a lot that be can to done to redress the balance and keep both of you sexually and emotionally satisfied. But there's one crucial piece of advice which makes all the difference here: you must stop blaming each other. So before we go any further, I want you to make a pact. Say it out loud to yourself in front of the mirror:

The way you treat each other out of bed, strongly impacts on how you'll be treated in it

'I will not blame my partner or punish them for who they are.' Then say it directly to them, 'I won't blame or punish you for who you are.' (Possibly fill them in on why you're telling them this or they might think you're referring to that nasty habit they have of picking their nose while you're not looking.) If you can do this – and keep reminding yourself of it – the rest is easy. The way you treat each other out of bed, strongly impacts on how you'll be treated in it. Each pulling back the covers with a vicious tug – the result of a day spent stewing resentfully over the problem – isn't getting either of you anywhere. The nicer you are and the more understanding you are out of bed, the quicker you'll see results in it.

I've divided the following into two sections – for those with high sex drive and those with low libido – but I want you to read both to get a better understanding of how the other feels.

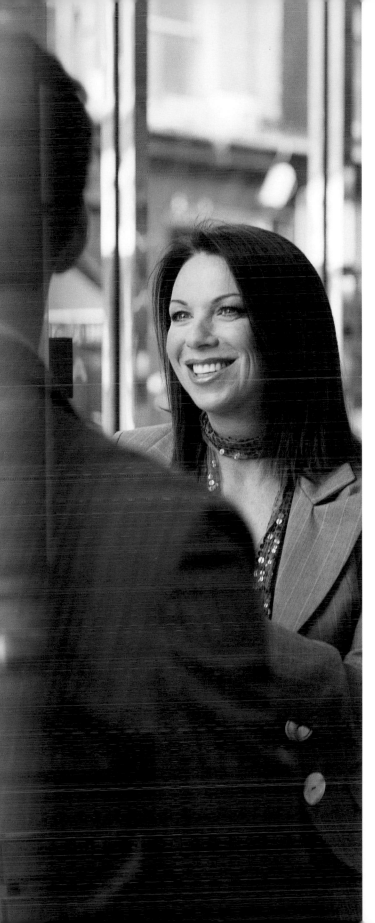

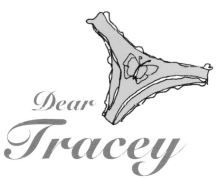

Dear *Tracey*

I WAS SO EAGER TO IMPRESS MY NEW BOYFRIEND, I FAKED ORGASM BECAUSE I DIDN'T WANT TO UPSET HIM. WHAT NOW?

We've all done it. And most of us do it when you did – right at the start, when we're auditioning for Potential Long-Term Girlfriend. We want to make sex perfect, so he'll see us as perfect and perfect sex, of course, includes an orgasm for both of you. Thing is though, while it may achieve what you want in the beginning – he falls in love and you end up staying together long-term – you're now in a bit of a pickle. Unless you confess at some point, you've effectively set yourself up for a lifetime of orgasm-less sex (not fun by anyone's standards). Faking it at any point doesn't do you or him any favours. It's not just pointless to fake it, it's disrespectful. It means you don't believe the person you are with is capable of giving you the ultimate in sexual pleasure. What to do now? I wouldn't make a big deal of it by confessing, I'd simply stop faking it from now on. Show him how you like to be touched by gently guiding his hands or tongue to the places you want them and give lots of positive feedback.

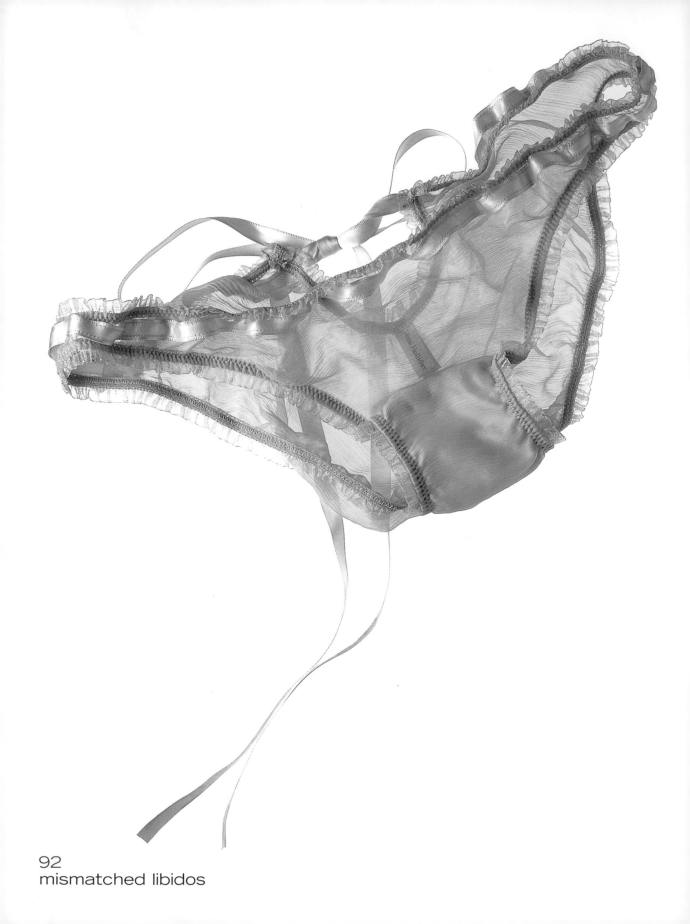

92
mismatched libidos

Things which can stop you feeling *Sexy*

EXHAUSTION, PROBLEMS WITH YOUR RELATIONSHIP: FEELING RESENTFUL, FRUSTRATED, SAD, EMPTY, GUILTY, ASHAMED, *stress,* LOW SELF-ESTEEM, *Poor general health,* BAD BODY IMAGE, TOO MUCH ALCOHOL, POOR SEX EDUCATION, *too many party drugs,* SOME PRESCRIBED MEDICATIONS, A TRAUMATIC SEXUAL EXPERIENCE (LIKE RAPE, ABUSE), DEPRESSION, *lack of trust,* LOW HORMONE LEVELS, MENOPAUSE, *periods,* PREGNANCY, A BAD LOVER, COMMUNICATION PROBLEMS, A HISTORY OF UNSATISFACTORY SEX, UNATTRACTIVE PARTNER, *partner has bad hygiene,* PELVIC SURGERY WHICH CAN DEADEN NERVE ENDINGS, ZERO CHEMISTRY, A STRICT, RELIGIOUS UPBRINGING

the 'I'd much rather
have a cup of tea' brigade

WHY DON'T I FEEL LIKE SEX? is a question most often asked by women – but that's because it's a lot harder for a man to own up to feeling that way. We (as in society) expect women (delicate, ladylike and ultra sensitive creatures, after all) to be a bit 'above' all that sort of thing.

Public perception doesn't have the average female half-crazed and rabid with lust when offered a sneaky glimpse of a naked foot. That's a man, silly! We (society) think of men as having voracious sexual appetites, permanently erect penises and a radar capable of spotting a 36DD from six miles away. As a man, having to admit you'd rather clean out the back shed than shag the missus – that's hard (even if the other bits aren't). So, let's clear up one myth immediately: not all women have low libidos, not all men have high libidos. It's a mix of both.

How the sexes do appear to differ in desire issues, however, is in what sparks it. While there will still be plenty of women who fall into the male camp and vice versa, there is a pretty consistent theme which experts are calling 'the intimacy trap'. Basically, women need love in order to want sex and men need sex in order to feel loved. (The problem's been around forever but experts are only just determining what to do about it!) What makes lots of women feel loved is talking.

Words are aphrodisiacs to us: we're very likely to feel like sex after a long, intense, emotional chat. What makes men feel loved is physical contact. A touch, kiss, a quick grab: these are his aphrodisiacs. Talking, to a lot of men, doesn't come easily. They find it difficult to do and many think it spoils intimate moments, rather than adds to them. With one sex wanting one thing, the other wanting something completely different, is it a case of 'never the twain shall meet'? Thankfully, there are things you can do to fix this (we're about to talk about that now) but simply being aware of each other's motives and needs helps enormously.

Women are very likely to feel like sex after a long, emotional chat

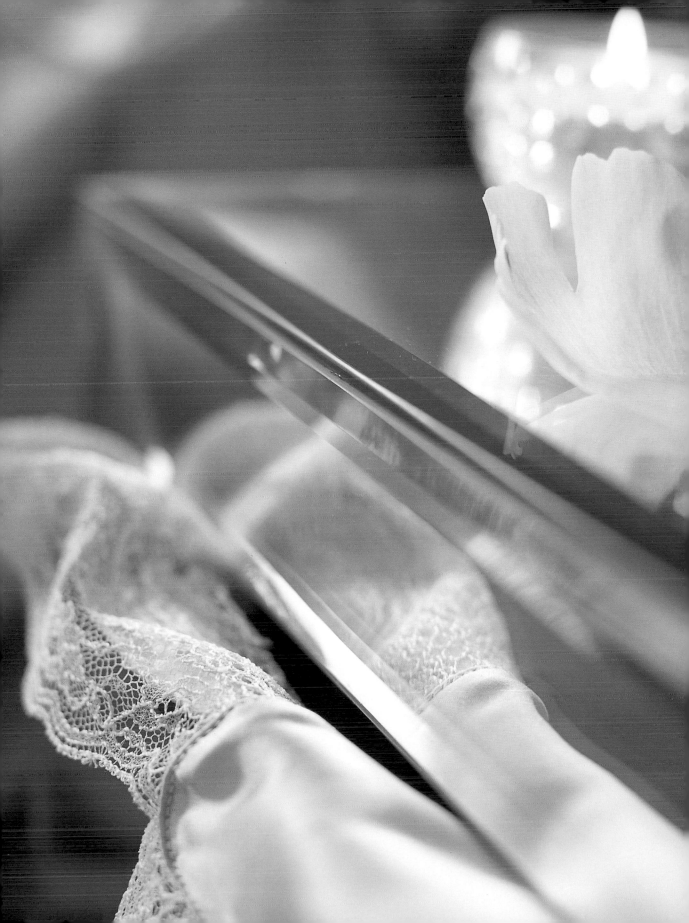

Things
you can do to even things up

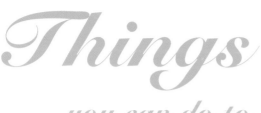

ACT ON IMPULSES

There's new evidence to suggest you'll never feel desire as strongly as your higher-sexed partner does – which means it's pointless waiting for it to happen. Highly sexed people report dramatic stirrings in the belly (not to mention other places) when feeling hot and bothered. Lower sexed people say that even at their highest peak, it feels more like a burning coal than a raging fire. If this is true, it makes sense for you to have sex at the 'flicker' stage, rather than waiting for the fire to develop. It might just go out instead!

3 ACCEPT RESPONSIBILITY

'I don't mind that he has a low sex drive,' said one of our healthily horny female contributors on *The Sex Inspectors*, 'But I do mind that he refuses to do anything about it, other than expect me to put up with it'. While it's true the person with the low libido is often seen as the 'cause' of the problem, it's also true they tend to set the pace for the amount of sex in the relationship. It's hard even for the highly sexed to keep desire raging over a long period. So don't just expect it to tap you on the shoulder, be proactive! Take responsibility for creating desire by figuring out what triggers it for you.

INCREASE YOUR SEXUAL IQ

Increase your sexual IQ. The more you understand about your body's desire cycle (see Chapter One), the more chance you have of working out what triggers a response. We're programmed to have sex, not satisfying sex. Mother Nature will instinctively guide you to the point where you'll help her make you pregnant but she's not terribly fussed if you enjoy the process or not. Knowledge is power. Gather a library of sex books and read them.

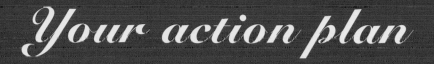

Your action plan

● VISIT YOUR DOCTOR to check your general health and review any medications which could be affecting your desire level.

● KEEP A SEX DIARY Write down any erotic thoughts and what triggers them. Keep track of how you're going with any of the techniques suggested here. The more you know about your responses, the better able you are to manipulate them.

● MAKE SURE YOUR ORGASM TRIGGER IS PARTNER FRIENDLY If you can only orgasm by lying face-down on a bed, using a piece of silk to rub yourself (cue Charlotte, one of our most famous Sex Inspector contributors), you're making it rather difficult for your partner to replicate.

● MAKE TIME FOR SOLVING THE PROBLEM Set aside time for trying things which could work (taking a bath, reading a sexy book). If you've got kids, don't use them as an excuse. I know it's hard but try not to resign as wife and become Mum only.

● DON'T SAY NO, SAY WHEN If you refuse sex, give some idea of when it's next on the agenda. There's a huge difference between 'No' and 'I don't feel like it now but I know I will tomorrow morning'.

● REJECT SEX, NOT THE PERSON Say 'I don't feel like sex, but I do feel like cuddling you because I love you so much.' It's infinitely preferable to pushing the person away and rolling over.

● HAVE SEX EVEN IF YOU DON'T REALLY FANCY IT Lots of people enjoy sex once they get started and there's evidence regular sex boosts the body's production of testosterone – which will make you feel like it more in future.

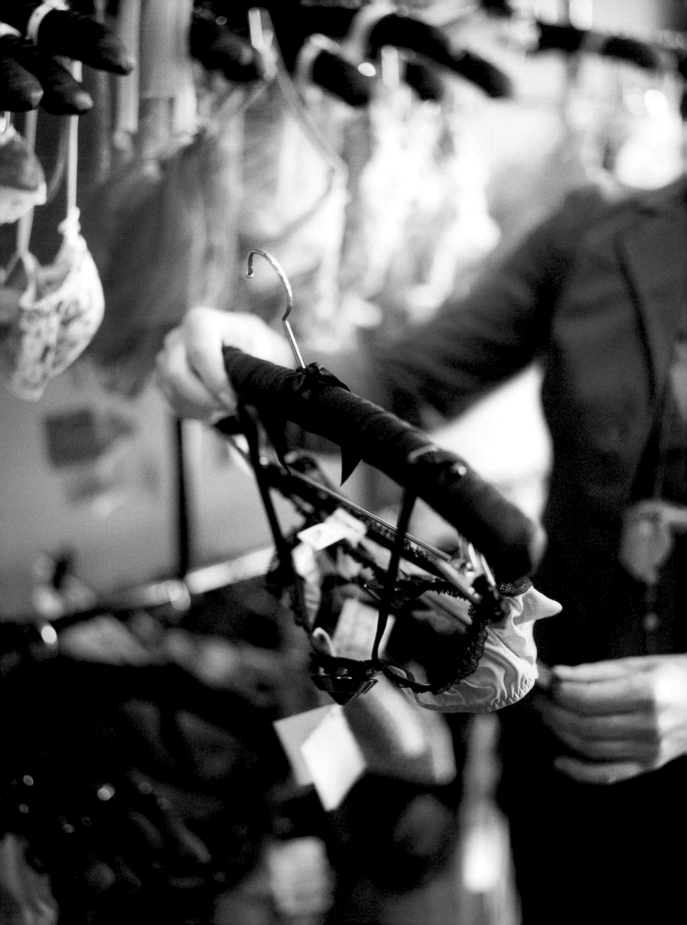

anywhere – anytime people

BECACAUSE SEX TO HIGH DESIRE PEOPLE is an extraordinarily exquisite experience they don't quite believe anyone wouldn't want to do it. So their resentment at being denied sex doesn't just come from not getting enough of what they want; it comes from feeling like they're being deliberately punished. Not able to understand the reason why sex wouldn't be top of the Thing I'd Most Like to Do Today (Now/This Second) list, they secretly believe low desire people do want sex – just not with them. This makes them feel unattractive, undesirable and ultimately not wanted when their partner says no. If you're a woman and being refused, you'll usually decide it must be because: a. you're too fat; b. someone cute has started at his work; c. your thighs are too fat; d. your bottom's too big. Guys tend to assume she's: a. been to one too many male stripper nights; or

It doesn't feel great being constantly knocked back and it dents even the toughest ego

b. fancies the cute new guy at work (strangely, few look down and blame their beer belly). Either way, it doesn't feel great being constantly knocked back and it dents even the toughest ego. All of us like to feel irresistible – especially to the person we love. You want to feel you're able to give someone sexual pleasure, rather than be a sexual pain in the ass. The first piece of advice for you: don't take it personally. Pretty well all of the time it doesn't mean your partner doesn't find you attractive; just that they don't find sex that attractive. There's plenty you can do to ease the situation – start by trying the following:

Things
you can do to even things up

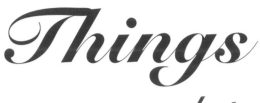

1 MASTURBATE MORE OFTEN

Ironically, this is recommended for both high and low libido people. Masturbating helps to increase desire but also takes the edge off if you're about to climb the walls. It's sometimes a good idea to masturbate an hour or so before you do have sex, if you find you're orgasming too quickly when you finally do get to do it.

3 SPEND 2 DAYS IN THEIR SHOES

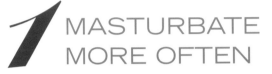

If you're at work and she's at home looking after the kids, imagine how you'd feel washing, cleaning, constantly having to be at someone else's beck and call. As you indulge in a pleasant five-minute daydream, she's coping with a screaming baby. Or vice versa. Some people thrive on parenting or working from home while their partner is on the work treadmill feeling trapped and unin-spired. By pretending you're them, you'll get a better idea of why they don't feel sexy or sexual. Try to imagine what it would be like if you didn't enjoy being touched, masturbating or having sex with your partner. Desire is an effortless, magical thing to the highly sexed. Low desire people really have to work at it.

UP THE AMOUNT OF NON-SEXUAL CONTACT

Kiss, hug and touch your partner as much as possible, but first agree on a signal which clearly says, 'This gesture is romantic, not sexual.' It might be that you agree to certain 'sex-free' days or periods of the day. One of the main problems of mismatched libidos is affection misinterpretation. You're too scared to touch them because when you do you're accused of harassing, and they're too scared to touch you in case you take it as an invitation for sex. The result – no touching – drives you even further apart.

Your action plan

● DON'T HASSLE THEM FOR SEX The best option of all, while you're trying out all these options, is to avoid initiating sex completely. Leave them to explore their various options, minus any pressure to perform, and let reverse psychology do its stuff. If it's up to them to initiate, suddenly they're in the power position.

● DON'T SULK WHEN THEY REFUSE SEX If you initiate and it's obvious they're not interested in following through, be gracious about it. Don't get all huffy, give them the silent treatment or a hard time. Just because you feel like sex at that moment, doesn't mean they have to. You're not interlinked computer systems, you're human beings!

● DO IT YOURSELF It's perfectly acceptable to want to masturbate if you're aroused and your partner's not interested in stimulating you. You could do it in front of them – they might be happy to indulge you in non-participatory sex (you masturbate while they watch) – but some find it just increases the guilt. Very obviously stomping off into the bathroom has the same effect. Talk it through with your partner. Where can you go to pleasure yourself without upsetting them?

● WHEN THEY DO ENJOY SEX, PAY ATTENTION What time of day is it? What had they been doing before? Who/how was it suggested? Are you doing anything differently? Try to pinpoint reasons as to why it's working that time but not others. You can then time your advances for when they're most likely to be welcomed.

● BECOME THEIR IDEA OF A GREAT LOVER, NOT YOURS Your idea of sexual nirvana may be their idea of hell. The more they enjoy sex with you, the more they'll want to do it. It's in your interest to appeal to their way of thinking, not yours.

supersexy solutions
(for both of you)

ONCE YOU'VE ACCEPTED responsibility for your own libido levels and implemented the 'action plans', it's time to come together again. You might find any or all of the following helpful.

A SEX CONTRACT

WHY IT WORKS: If you're arguing over how much sex you have or what type of sex you have, this will work for you. It allows you a let's-sort-it-all-out-NOW solution as opposed to something you need to argue over daily, feeling resentful and put-upon.

PROPS YOU'LL NEED: An A4 notepad, pen and paper.

HOW IT WORKS: Head two separate pages with: 'The amount of sex I'd like' and 'The type of sex I'd like', and draw a line down the middle, one side for each of you. Now, each take turns in detailing what you want. Start with the quantity of sex you'd each like over a two-month period (it's too restrictive to do it weekly or monthly). At one end put an 'in my dreams' total of sessions per week; at the other end put the 'I guess I could live with' total. Do the same with the 'type of sex I'd like'. In this, you're providing details on how long you want the session to last, what it would involve (oral, intercourse, mutual masturbation, fantasy, roleplay, whatever else takes your fancy) and one adjective to sum up the mood (lusty, romantic, etc). This not only helps your partner know what you like, it focuses you on what you'd like. Think about the best time of the day/week to have sex, who initiates, add in non-sexual things (stroking, cuddles, kissing, head, shoulder and body massages). Once you've finished this part of the exercise you have – literally, spelt out in black and white – a sexual wishlist of what each of you would like in an ideal world, and what each is willing to settle for. Now, you're ready to barter. Head up another sheet called 'Our Sex Life for the Next Two Months'. You're aiming for compromises but it's not just about settling in the middle. If you want sex six times a week but your partner wants it three, you might be happy with fewer sessions if one of them lasts an hour or so and the quicker sessions are lusty rather than lack-lustre.

It's an ideal sexual wishlist of what each of you would like

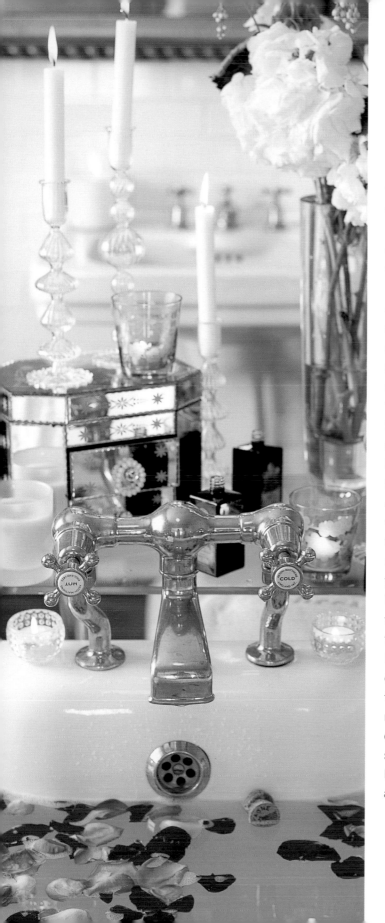

WHAT NOW? The Sex Contract works for lots of couples because it stops you second-guessing each other: spontaneity works for some people, others like to know exactly what's expected of them. It also sets clear boundaries for couples who are scared to receive or show affection for fear of it being misinterpreted. When I suggest this exercise some couples resist it because they don't like the concept of bartering for sex but, however unromantic, relationships are all about give and take. I see nothing wrong with making love to your partner when you're not frothing at the mouth for it yourself, because you know damn well they indulged you the week before when you were dying for it and they were a bit lukewarm. So long as it's done with an attitude of sexual generosity (you did that for me, so I'm doing this for you) rather than resentment (you didn't bother doing that for me, so why should I do this for you?), I consider 'bartering' perfectly acceptable.

2 THE MAGNET METHOD

WHY IT WORKS: If your problem is more a frequency mismatch, this simple system works a treat. As with the sex contract, the main aim is to stop the 'Do they/don't they want sex?' daily dilemma which has both of you circling each other, sniffing the air for clues. It requires zero effort and it's great for couples who don't feel comfortable discussing their sexual needs (you'd still be far better off if you did, mind you!).

PROPS YOU'LL NEED: Two fridge magnets, easily distinguishable from each other. (If you don't have a fridge, use something you can each pin on a noticeboard.)

HOW IT WORKS: Each of you should claim a magnet, then move it once a day depending on whether you do or don't feel like sex. If the magnet is close to the top of the fridge, it means you're extremely interested. If it's at the bottom, you'd rather be put on the Cabbage Soup Diet for life. There's a temptation for the high sex person to leave their magnet at the top of the fridge permanently and the low-desire person to weld theirs to the bottom, but you're actually better off doing the opposite. If both of you try to resist your 'natural' inclination and deliberately hover in neutral territory (the middle of the fridge), you might find an interesting pattern emerges. The low-desire person – albeit nervously and tentatively – (finally) gets to be the first to instigate sex by inching their magnet above the always-up-for-it person, experiencing an hypnotic twinge of sexual power. The high-desire person (finally) gets the equally exquisite glory of being seduced.

WHAT NOW? Some couples keep the magnets on the fridge forever, others find after a few months it's removed the pressure to the point where they're happy verbalizing their needs.

THE SENSATE FOCUS PROGRAMME

WHY IT WORKS: It's used regularly by sex therapists to reawaken desire when your libido is low. (It's also useful if you spent all your life getting carried away by the sensation of sex – and who could blame you! – without really paying attention to what was actually being done, where and when to you. It's only later, when you're in a long-term relationship, that this information is crucial.) The idea is to reawaken sexual feelings gradually, using a form of self- and partner massage to learn how to give and receive pleasure.

PROPS YOU'LL NEED: A private place where you won't be disturbed. A bath or shower. Gel, shower or body oil. Body moisturizer and massage oil.

HOW IT WORKS: As you're following the programme, it's crucial to concentrate on the sensations you're experiencing, rather than try to analyse why you're feeling what you're feeling or anticipate what's going to happen next.

● You can do this naked in bed or while having a bath or shower. Begin by massaging yourself all over. Start at the top of your head and work down, experimenting with different strokes (soft, firm, fast, slow). Focus on the now and think about nothing but what feels good and arouses you. Don't just concentrate on genitals and breasts but all your body – every square inch of it.

● Now you're going to do the same to your partner and have them do the same to you. Set the scene (soothing music, muted lighting) then take turns massaging each other, top to toe,

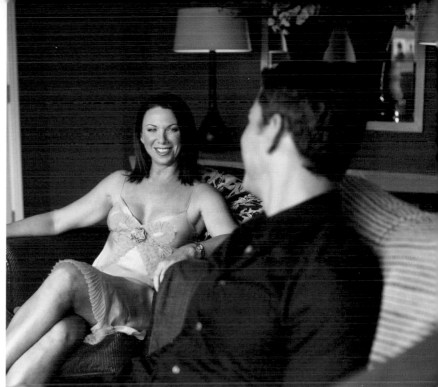

The idea is to reawaken sexual feelings gradually, using a self and partner massage

front and back (but avoid the obvious sexual zones like breasts and genitals). As you're being massaged, give your partner feedback by providing a running commentary on what feels good and what doesn't. Before you start, make a pact with each other that you won't be offended by honesty (for instance, a certain touch may not feel as great as your partner has always believed!)

● Same as above, except you're now allowed to move onto the naughty bits. But you're officially allowed to touch more sexually sensitive parts with one proviso: you must continue to talk constantly and keep up a running commentary of what stroke and pressure feels best. After you've finished touching, try kissing and licking. Only when you've explored each stage thoroughly, and both of you feel ready, do you have permission to have intercourse.

WHAT NOW? The idea of sensate focus is to take you and your partner right back to basics, removing all preconceived ideas of what you like/don't like. It officially works to awaken desire in low libido people but is equally effective at reacquainting the bored and desensitized with sexual feelings.

Things which can keep you **Horny**

EXERCISE, SHOWING OFF A FIT, TONED BODY, *fresh air*, SUNSHINE, LAUGHTER, A HEALTHY SOCIAL LIFE, ALCOHOL IN MODERATION, ***not smoking***, GOOD PERSONAL HYGIENE, CHOCOLATE (IT CONTAINS THEOBROMINE WHICH BOOSTS ENDORPHINS), *the right amount of sleep*, FOODS HIGH IN OMEGA-3 (SEXUAL AROUSAL): FISH, NUTS, FOODS HIGH IN ZINC (SEXUAL AROUSAL AND FERTILITY): SHELLFISH, EGGS, CHEESE, CHICKEN, BROWN RICE, FOODS HIGH IN IRON (AROUSAL): RED MEAT, CHICKEN, EGGS, SPINACH, PULSES, *foods high in magnesium (sexual stamina): green leafy vegetables, nuts, bananas*, FOODS HIGH IN VITAMIN B (ENERGY): WHOLEGRAINS, NUTS, MEAT, FISH, EGGS, **FEELING HAPPY,** ATTRACTIVE CLOTHES, *sex,* MASTURBATION, A WELCOMING BEDROOM, EROTIC BOOKS AND DVDS, WEEKENDS AWAY, TIME TO RELAX

what if both of us are happy not having sex?

IF YOU'RE BOTH PUSHING ninety and need a Zimmer frame to move around in bed, you're officially allowed to give up on sex. I also acknowledge there are couples out there where both partners have zero or extremely low libidos and seriously aren't bothered by a future which doesn't include any sex. So good luck to the twenty or so couples under sixty, world-wide, who truly do fall into this category. The thing is, the chances of finding and hooking up with someone who has exactly the same sex drive as you is extremely rare. Even couples who pride themselves on having evenly matched desire levels can point to discrepancies when pushed: one inevitably fancying it more than the other in certain situations. Which means, in my opinion, pretty much everyone who stops having sex is risking their relationship.

Let me explain. We get more from sex than we think. Not only does it keep us physically satisfied, it provides much-needed excitement and stimulation in our lives.

Sex makes us feel wanted and attractive, needed and admired. We feel emotionally connected to the person we're having sex with. Touching and orgasm release endorphins (feel-good chemicals) which create a feeling of well-being. Satisfying sex also boosts our immune system and promotes production of a substance called oxytocin, making us feel warm and snuggly. Because it makes our blood pump furiously, sex is good for the heart in a physical sense, but also in an emotional capacity. Humans are driven to seek pleasure and sex encourages our body to release the pleasure substance, PEA (phenylethylamine), making us feel light-headed and light-hearted. Sex reduces stress and frustration levels, makes our skin glow, our hair shine and our eyes sparkle.

It's easy to forget how good sex is and how all of the above feels, when you're not getting any. But there will come a time when you're reminded of how good it was. You're away on a

We get more from sex than we think. Not only does it keep us physically satisfied, it provides much needed excitement in our lives

conference, working late, and the friendly, attractive waiter leans forward to clear your food away and you get a whiff of his aftershave and out of nowhere, suddenly you remember and all those memories of hot, frantic, fabulous sex rush back at alarming speed. Even sexed-up couples feel the pull of 'Why not?' in situations like this. How are you or your partner going to cope when you've not only been starved of sex (even if voluntarily), you/they know having their appetite reawakened means little because the bored-with-sex partner at home hasn't had the same experience. Yes, you could try racing home and saying, 'Honey, I remember how great sex was! Let's do it up against the wall like we used to!' But if you honestly think that'll be greeted with a yawn, disapproving frown and 'I thought we discussed we weren't doing that anymore' sniff, you might well opt to chat up the

An attractive waiter leans forward to clear your food away ... suddenly you remember all those hot, frantic, fabulous sex sessions

dishy waiter/waitress instead. Or work colleague. Or that guy/girl on the bus who you've started chatting to lately, feeling an oddly familiar stirring below as you do so. No matter how much your partner loves you, no matter how much they or you believe they're immune to temptation, they're not. And you're not. Stop having sex with each other and you risk both of you wanting to have sex with someone else. It's that simple. So if your excuse for not 'doing it' is simply that neither of you feel like it anymore because you've been together 'forever' and it seems like 'such an effort' and you'd both 'really honestly rather watch telly together', perhaps you might like to have a little rethink.

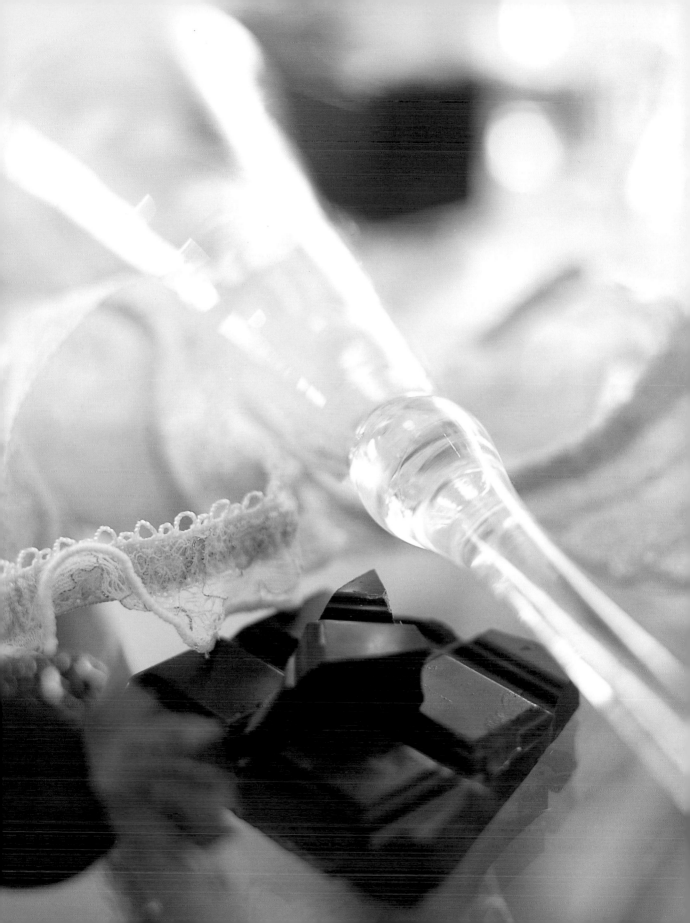

guys – want more sex?
do more housework

OK, I'M UNASHAMEDLY directing this section to men because, sad as it is, I've heard few complaints from men about their partners not doing their portion of the housework. But I have met a staggering amount of women who admit they withheld sex because their partner wasn't too hot at helping with the dishes. Men not sharing domestic chores is a major cause of resentment in relationships. And her feeling resentful means one thing: less or no sex. The quickest way for you to boost the amount of sex you're having is to do your share of the housework. Don't panic, you don't need to turn into Mrs Doubtfire, just a fair, considerate person. Here are a few hints to help you along the way:

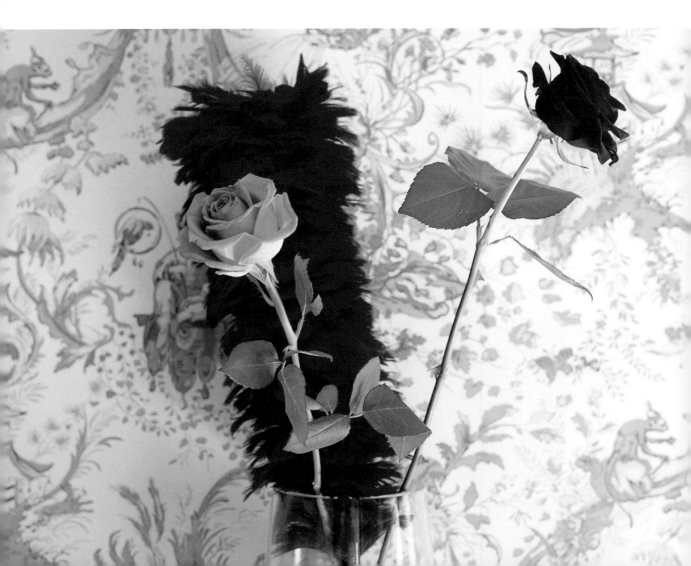

Change your attitude...

HOUSEWORK ISN'T 'WOMAN'S WORK', IT'S A COUPLE'S JOB. YOU BOTH CREATE THE MESS, IT'S LOGICAL BOTH OF YOU SHOULD CLEAN IT UP. YOU AREN'T 'HELPING' BY DOING THE DISHES, YOU'RE SHARING THE NECESSARY CHORES WHICH MAKE BOTH YOUR LIVES MORE COMFORTABLE.

Make friends with Jamie Oliver

If you're not already doing some of the cooking (and loads of men are, which is great), give it a go. Otherwise, once the chores are divided up, you'll be stuck with all the really boring bits like hoovering (yuk), ironing (YUK!). Believe me, cooking is fun compared to cleaning the loo.

THINK OUTSIDE THE BOX

In some situations, it makes sense for one person to shoulder the lion's share of the housework. If she's not working right now or only working part-time, it makes sense for her to do more than you. If your job's a breeze and she's working all hours to get that promotion, it's fairer for you to shoulder a bigger portion. Some couples take turns week by week. Others – very sensibly in my book – hire a cleaner and spend their precious time off having fun and having sex. You can also use trade-offs. She might put up with doing all the washing and ironing if you give her two weekly massages. The bottom line as always: compromise and communication.

Blame your mum

If you come from a home where Mum mothered Dad, you're eighty per cent more likely to think housework and fussing over someone is what females do. Thing is, though, your Mum probably worked full-time as a housewife whereas your wife probably holds down a job as well as looking after you.

THE MORE HOUSEWORK YOU DO, THE BETTER SEX LIFE YOU'LL HAVE

Both sex and housework require energy, and most of us have only got so much left of it at the end of a hard day. Think about what you do when you come home from work. Do you flop in front of the telly while she organizes dinner, cooks, cleans up, does the dishes and works out what's needed for tomorrow night's meal? Well, surprise, surprise – guess who's going to feel more like sex when they get into bed? If you do your bit, she'll not only have more energy left for sex, she'll feel more valued and respected. Her head will feel like sex as well as her body because she will like you more!

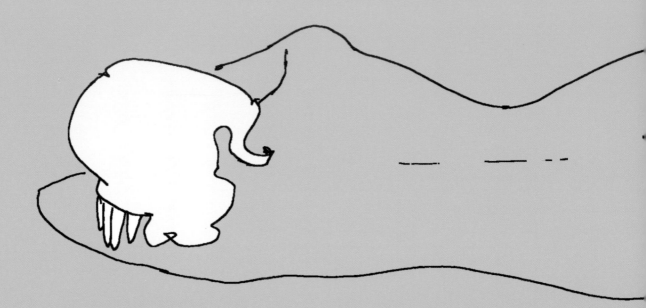

the
female
orgasm

Why she needs more than just
your penis to orgasm and other
must-know facts about female
satisfaction

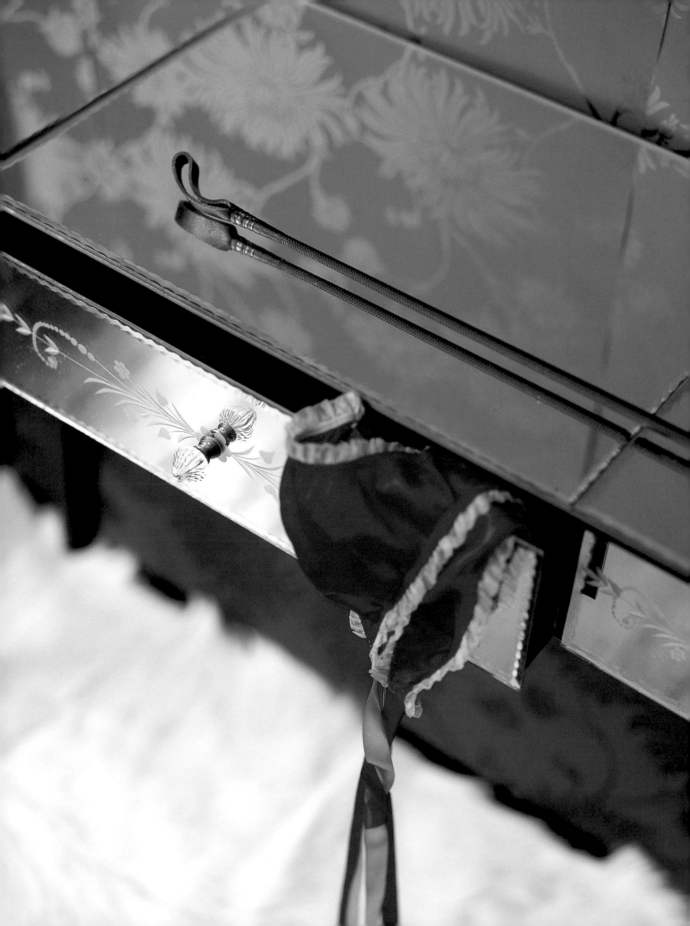

*L*ESS THAN THIRTY PER CENT OF WOMEN ORGASM THROUGH INTERCOURSE and half of those are probably faking. There, I said it! Now guys, when you're through banging the table (with your fist that is), puffing your chest out and indignantly/smugly thinking 'Well, Susie sure as hell never did!! And if that (little lady) was faking, well, she should be up for an Oscar!' listen up. You might learn something. Fact is, I agree with you – the bit about the Oscar anyway. I'm sure Susie did a fine acting job. As do millions of women just like her. Every single day.

Which begs an obvious question: if women not climaxing through intercourse alone is such a common problem, why are we all lying about it? You can understand men wanting to believe the hype – after all, they're the owners of the penis (whose image suffers somewhat from all this). But why would women collaborate to support a lie which is not only clearly false but interfering with our ultimate pleasure?

It goes something like this …

Susie lied because she loved her boyfriend and was worried he wouldn't like her as much if she didn't orgasm when he expected her to.

Susie also lied to her close girlfriends during a spill-all-the-secrets-along-with-the-alcohol girls-night-out. She was going to confess but then Jayne started boasting how she came every single time and Susie certainly didn't want to look bad in front of her!

In reality, Jayne wasn't boasting, she was actually testing the water to see if anyone else might challenge her. Because they didn't, she now assumes she's the only one in the group who's 'not normal'. So she continues moaning and groaning and 'doing a Meg', so her boyfriend Jake remains none the wiser.

When Jayne and Jake split, he meets Jessica and assumes she'll be able to orgasm via penetration because Jayne did. When (brave, honest) Jessica confesses she can't – and never has – he tells her this has never happened to him before. Although he quite liked Jessica, Jake's not sure it makes him feel terribly sexy being with someone who clearly doesn't feel the same about him. Because if she did enjoy having intercourse with him, she'd climax right? After all, everyone else does! And so Jake dumps Jessica and he meets Kate and out comes the whole sad story of how his ex Jessica didn't. Kate thinks, 'Brave girl, that Jessica,' but she's no fool and she likes Jake a lot, so she assures him she doesn't have any problems in that department. Why would she? And so it continues…

Most women don't faint at the sight of a throbbing erection

The way to make men understand most women don't faint and/or climax at the sight of a throbbing erection (however fabulous that sight might be), and for women to understand it's okay not to be in raptures over a few thrusts (however well-aimed), is for us all to stick to the same story. Present a united front. So let's give it a go. Here it is in in BIG letters so you can let it imprint indelibly on your brain:

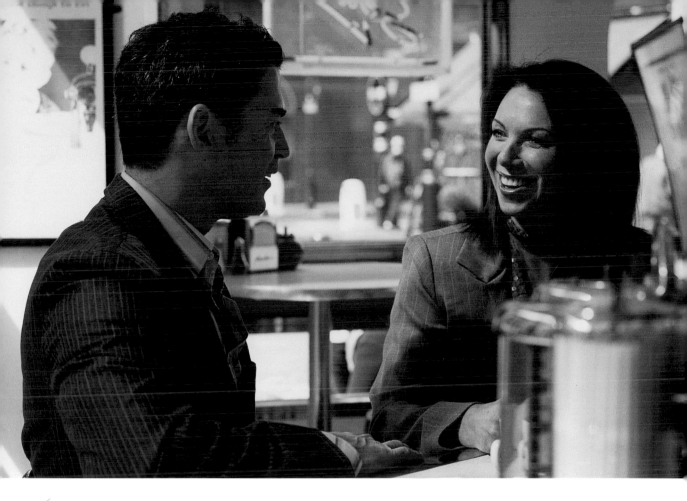

'AROUND THREE QUARTERS OF WOMEN DON'T ORGASM THROUGH INTERCOURSE. PENETRATION ALONE IS RARELY EVER ENOUGH'

As a former Associate Editor of Cosmopolitan magazine, I can tell you the number one reader question is, 'How can I have an orgasm during intercourse?' And I know for a fact that editors world-wide concur. This chapter is devoted to helping women achieve their full potential – but mainly to the men who honestly want to understand them. Put aside all those preconceptions and take a deep breath.

The hard evidence

I don't care how many ex or current girlfriends' groans you want to cite as evidence, chances are your partner isn't satisfied simply by your penis alone. (Sorry Wilbur) If you don't want to believe me, take a tip from the following prominent sexperts:

● **THE BERMAN TWINS,** US sexologists, bluntly state, 'most women don't have orgasms with intercourse alone.'

● **UK SEXPERT SUZI GODSON** acknowledges eighty per cent of women who can achieve orgasm can't do it without clitoral stimulation. She also cites a study which shows only 28.6 per cent of women experience orgasm with regular sex partners.

● **UK SEX THERAPIST BERNIE ZILBERGELD SAYS,** 'It's now widely accepted that clitoral stimulation is what leads to orgasm in most women.'

● **US CLINICAL SEXOLOGIST IAN KERNER SAYS,** 'All orgasms are clitoral. The clitoris is the sexual epicenter, an orgasm powerhouse.' He also cites a study which suggests the G-spot may be nothing more than the back end of the clitoris, since its roots run so deep.

● **EM AND LO, FOUNDERS OF THE EDGY NERVE.COM,** put it beautifully in their book The Big Bang: 'For guys, the formula of intercourse ecstasy is usually fairly simple: insert dick, thrust some more, come. Unfortunately, only the rare, lucky woman who likes cervical stimulation will get off from this equation. And guys: you're probably not dating one of them. How to achieve simultaneous orgasm during penetration every time? We have no idea.'

● **DR CAROLE ALTMAN, A HIGHLY RESPECTED AMERICAN SEX THERAPIST, SAYS,** 'I feel it unnecessary to go deeply into the great argument about the vaginal vs the clitoral orgasm. There is only one orgasm and that is achieved through clitoral stimulation.'

● **KINSEY, ONE OF THE WORLD'S BEST KNOWN SEX RESEARCHERS,** acknowledged in his original 1950s findings that more than half of all women required clitoral stimulation to orgasm. In the Kinsey New Edition (1990), it's acknowledged some researchers have upped this figure to seventy-five per cent.

so how do the
lucky ones do it?

THERE ARE SEVERAL THEORIES to explain how women have 'no hands' orgasms during intercourse (meaning no simultaneous finger stimulation of the clitoris). The obvious is that they're clearly witches who have done dastardly deals with the devil. One soul in return for a lifetime of easy orgasms? It's certainly tempting. But having spent years in Australia, I'm not such a fan of living in a hot climate. Other, less exciting explanations include:

● POSITION OR SIZE OF THE CLITORIS

Positions where the thrusting motion pulls down on the labia, are far more likely to get results because they're stimulating the clitoris. The larger your clitoris, the more chance it has of being 'rubbed'. If the clitoris is positioned lower than usual, closer to the vaginal entrance, this also increases the chance of 'accidental' stimulation.

● PRESSURE AGAINST THE CLITORAL AREA

Women who can orgasm purely through intercourse tend to press their pelvises against some part of the man, usually his pubic bone. This is the general theory behind the Coital Alignment Technique (page 123).

● VAGINAL RESPONSIVITY

Call it the 'G-spot' if you like, but there certainly appear to be particularly sensitive areas of the vagina which, when stimulated, produce orgasm. In almost all cases, the 'spots' the women refer to are on the front vaginal wall (though in totally different places on it, which puts paid to the G-spot hypothesis). The 'responsivity' theory is supported by the fact that the most successful 'no hands' orgasm positions cited are woman on top or rear-entry – the best positions for hitting the front wall.

look honey, no hands!

ARMED WITH THIS KNOWLEDGE, you'd be justified in thinking, 'Oh, sod it!' and deciding to stick with your tried-and-true formula of giving her an orgasm through oral sex, and him through intercourse. This, quite frankly, is what most couples tend to do. I hasten to point out here that just because lots of women don't have orgasms through intercourse, it doesn't mean they're not having a very nice time, thank you very much. Plenty report intense pleasure from feeling 'filled up'. Other comments include: 'It's incredibly bonding'; 'It's one hell of a turn on'; 'Watching his bottom go up and down is the sexiest sight in the world'; 'I might not climax but feeling him, rock hard, pumping into me, rockets me into a cerebral orgasm.' (And no, I didn't just include them to soothe any dented male egos, even though it's got to help!)

Apart from the first inch or so, the rest of the vagina receives little stimulation from the penis

Thing is, the skin of the inner vagina just isn't terribly sensitive. It's a thoughtful touch of Mother Nature to only put nerve endings (sensory perceptors) at the mouth of the vagina. Childbirth is excruciating enough without feeling it all the way down! This is also why the length of the penis isn't important: apart from the first inch or so, the rest of the vagina receives little stimulation from the penis. But while the inner two thirds are insensitive to touch, they are sensitive to pressure and stretch. This is why thrusting feels good, even if it doesn't produce orgasm.

Plenty of women also report feeling a distinct climbing then falling 'wave' of pleasure during intercourse, which feels a hell of a lot like

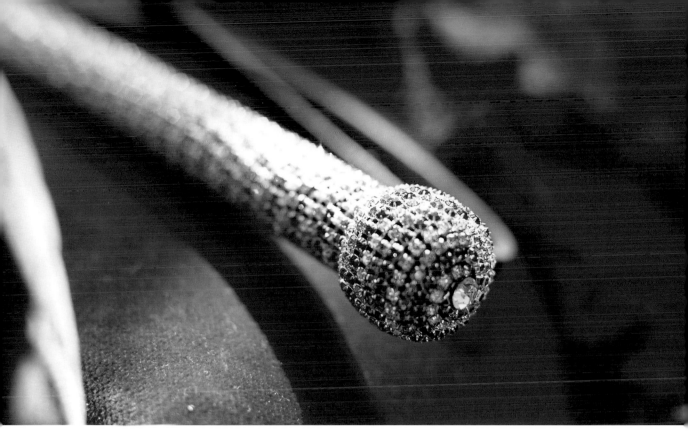

an orgasm. It lacks the distinct, sharp, intense contractions which accompany clitoral stimulation but it's certainly up there on the 'More Please!' scale. So deciding to stick with bog-standard intercourse and give in to Mother Nature's cruel little joke of putting the clitoris outside the vagina is totally acceptable. The 'she comes first (through oral) and he comes later (through intercourse)' technique has been around ever since humans learnt to put their tongues in places nature probably didn't intend.

But it's a bit wimpy, don't you think? Where's that fighting spirit, eh? Now you've both been reassured you're normal (amusing how we love being called that when it comes to sex and health results, but are insulted for anything else), how about refusing to be put into a box. Literally. The techniques below are designed to up your chances of having intercourse orgasms. If at first you don't succeed, try and try again because even if you don't achieve your original objective, I guarantee you'll have had damn good fun (and more than a few 'cheat' orgasms, if/when you've switched back to your old ways to tip over the edge). Good luck!

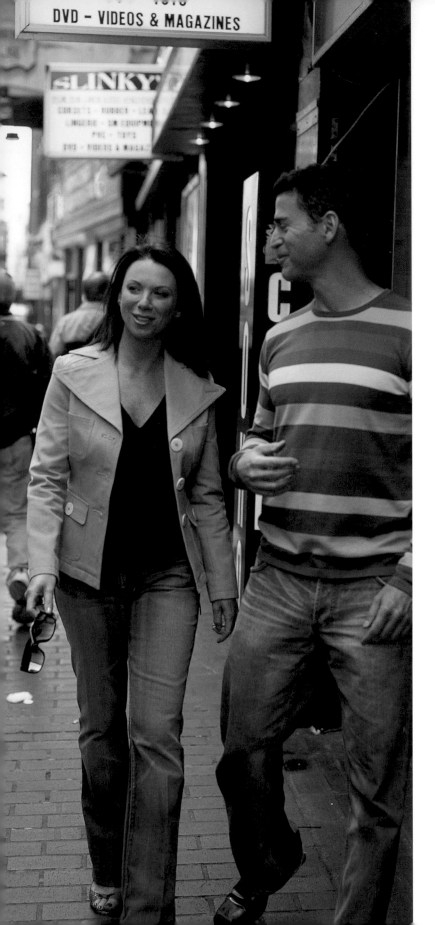

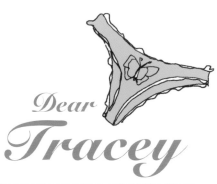

Dear *Tracey*

SOMETIMES I SEEM TO GET STUCK AT THE POINT JUST BEFORE ORGASM. AS MUCH AS IT FEELS NICE TO BE HOVERING AT THAT I-THINK-I'M-ABOUT-TO-BUT-THEN-AGAIN-MAYBE-NOT STAGE, GETTING STUCK THERE ISN'T AS MUCH FUN.

As well as trying all the tricks and tips listed in the chapter, try switching stimulation. You've probably desensitized yourself – done the same thing for so long, your body needs a kick to push it over the edge. Try adding something new. If you're into anal stimulation, a well-lubricated finger delivered with sensitivity and timing could do the trick. If that's not your cup of tea, try the old 'fake it till you make it' method. Pretend you're going into the throes of orgasm (clench your bottom and thighs, moan, throw your head back), and you may trick your body into doing just that by providing all the 'triggers' it associates with orgasm. Didn't work? Then change position. Get him to lie on his back, legs stretched out and together, then climb on top so you have complete control. Put your knees either side of his chest, let him penetrate and, leaning forward, move your hips in small circles so your clitoris makes contact with his pubic bone. It's also easy to climb off from here and move yourself upward: if his penis isn't doing it for you, his tongue might!

top 'tip-you-over' techniques

I'VE CALLED THEM 'TIP-YOU-OVER' TECHNIQUES because that's what women report back: they can sort of/almost/kind of get there through penetration but can't seem to jump over the line. These might just help you get to the other side.

FIRST PLACE
The CAT Technique

It's called CAT – the Coital Alignment Technique – and it's reputed to be the all-time best position for clitoral stimulation during intercourse. It's also a complicated, complex intercourse technique which requires real patience and persistence to get right because it means resisting the natural urge to thrust. Why bother if it's so bloody hard to master? Well, if this doesn't score you a 'no hands' intercourse orgasm, nothing will. (And you might even get a simultaneous one thrown in for good luck!) CAT is officially the brainchild of sexologist Edward Eichel. In the early nineties, he claimed to have discovered a brand new way to have sex which guaranteed orgasm for her – in the missionary position no less! – every time. While Eichel certainly didn't score Brownie points for modesty, he was generally applauded for at least trying to think outside the box. By taking the focus off internal stimulation (provided by thrusting) and concentrating instead on providing external stimulation (via pressure on the clitoris), he's definitely on the right track. This pressure/counterpressure technique is (of course) detailed in the Kama Sutra (what isn't in there?). Eichel, however, has simplified it, dazzled us with science – and come up with some pretty impressive statistics. At the start twenty-three per cent of women said they could orgasm through intercourse, and this jumped to seventy-seven per cent by the end.

Fancy giving it a try? Practise the basics with your clothes on, work on getting the rhythm right, then settle in for an average of five practice sessions before you start to really get the hang of it. I know, I know, it's not easy. But (believe me), it's worth making the effort.

If this doesn't score you a 'no-hands' intercourse orgasm, nothing will

BASIC POSITION He starts in the missionary position, penis inserted. Now he should move up her body a few inches (towards the head of the bed). His pelvis should be directly over hers with just the tip of his penis inside. The shaft is pressing against her mons.

LEGS His are together and straight. Hers are wrapped around his thighs, her ankles resting on his calves but more straight than bent.

UPPER BODY He cups her shoulders with his arms under her armpits so he's resting on her. His head is next to hers on the pillow. His upper body is totally relaxed, keep both your backs as straight as possible.

THE MOTION Forget in-out thrusting. This is a slow, rocking, hip action based on pressure and counterpressure. As one pushes, the other provides resistance. Full on direct penetration is impossible – but that's the point. Think external not internal stimulation. Think constant pressure on the clitoris.

HOW TO DO IT She tips her pelvis away from him and down into the bed. As she does so, his penis will slip out almost all the way, the base pressing against her clitoris. He now needs to move forward so his pelvis is three to four inches higher up her body. Remember, the head of the penis is just inside, the base is against her clitoris. Then it's his turn: he pushes down with his pelvis, so he moves lower down her body and penetrates fully. She tilts up to allow this to happen. Then it's her turn again. Keep repeating.

RHYTHM Don't speed up or slow down; instead maintain an even, steady pace. Why are vibrators so efficient at making women climax? Because they provide perfect consistent rhythm.

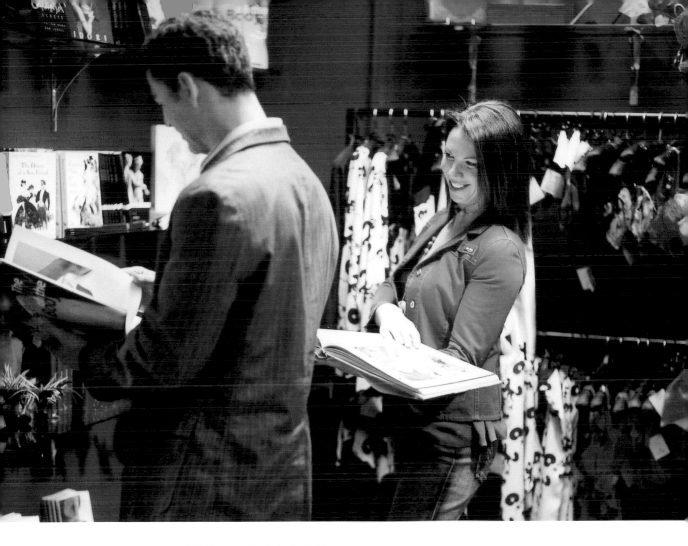

SECOND PLACE
The Bridge Technique

Adding a finger – yours or theirs – to stimulate the clitoris during intercourse is sometimes nicknamed the 'bridge' technique because it effectively provides a 'bridge' between his orgasm and hers. Pure penile stimulation might not work but by directly stimulating the clitoris during penetration, there's no reason why she can't orgasm while he's inside her. The trick is to use lots of lubricant and choose positions which allow one (or both of you) to use your fingers without getting cramps. Try woman on top (lean forward and lift up a little for easier access for him; or lean back and do-it-yourself); rear entry allows even easier access, as do face to face positions while sitting or kneeling.

A CLOSE THIRD
Adding a Vibrator

Some people find finger masturbation too much like hard work and (quite sensibly, in my opinion) opt for a small vibrator to do the job. Vibrators are a highly under-rated and under-used sex toy for couples. This is despite the fact that more UK women own one than own a washing machine! The reasons why they're the must-have bedroom accessory are many. They're quick – it's difficult for women not to orgasm while using a vibrator! And that's good news for couples whose libidos don't quite match because it takes the pressure off and there are bound to be times when you feel like sex and they don't (or vice versa). Single women also love them because if you can look after yourself, you're far less likely to start humping lamp-posts or that

The best vibrators for the job aren't penis-shaped but instead have a slightly rounded surface

really dodgy guy in the bar simply because you're desperate for a bit. The best vibrators for the job aren't penis-shaped but instead have a slightly rounded surface. Very few women (around fifteen per cent) insert things into the vagina when masturbating and – as evidenced by the theme of this entire chapter – the reason why is because most get their orgasms via external stimulation, not internal. Now women are becoming more involved with the design of vibrators, the ten-inch-throbbing-veined-just-like-the-real-thing versions are being phased out. Phew. Both women and men ran a mile when those were pulled out of the bedside drawer.

How to Use a Vibrator

● *Solo* Hold it firmly against the closed lips of the labia and vary the pressure (try rolling it around the area) until you orgasm. Some women stand up, some sit with legs apart, some lie down. Also try standing with your legs apart and holding the vibrator still in front of your genitals. You move backward and forward, grinding against it.

● *With your partner* Hold it against the side of your mouth while giving oral sex; press it lightly against his testicles or his or her perineum (the smooth bit between the bottom and testicles or vaginal opening). Most importantly, during intercourse, hold it against the clitoris for a no-fuss way to achieve penetrative orgasm.

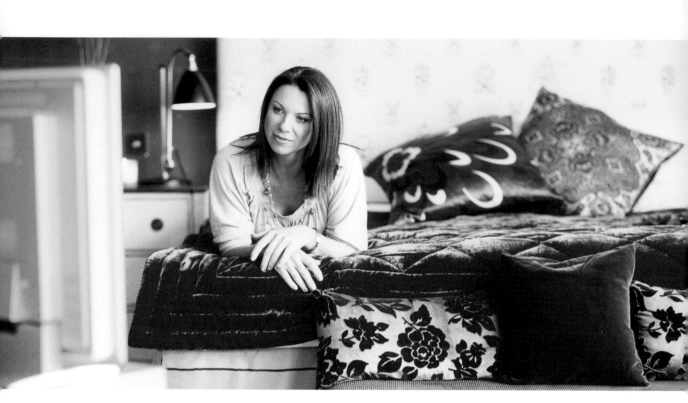

FOURTH PLACE
Hitting the Wall

While research on the G-spot has gone decidedly quiet, there's one thing most sex researchers and educators aren't disputing: that the front wall of the vagina is more sensitive than the rest. The reason why anyone's loath to settle on a specific area and name it after a letter of the alphabet, is because there's simply not enough evidence to support the original theory. German gynaecologist Ernest Grafenberg documented an area in the vagina which could induce orgasm and female ejaculation in 1950. His research fast got overshadowed by a focus on the clitoris (understandable, since it's easier to find, easier to manipulate and at least everyone has one!) but was revived by sexperts Whipple and Perry in 1981. In 2001, a New York researcher, Dr Terence Hines, kindly informed us that proof of the G-spot's existence (Grafenberg's study) was based on a mere dozen females and only four out of those twelve showed sensitivity. Which, let's face it, aren't exactly brilliant results.

Autopsies show no evidence of a G-spot, though advocates argue it's because it only appears when the person is aroused. Other 'evidence' suggests some people have a G-spot, some don't. While there's obviously some truth in the initial claim – as I said, there definitely is a particularly sensitive area that's stimulated by applying pressure to the front wall of the vagina – packing a picnic lunch and spotlight and refusing to return from the search unless victorious, could mean you're gone forever. It's worth exploring, however, in our quest for a penetrative orgasm. And anyway, who knows what other hotspots you might discover while rummaging around down there!

● FINGERS AND TOYS ARE MORE LIKELY TO HIT A G-SPOT than a penis and there are dildos and vibrators specifically designed for this purpose. They can reach further than fingers and are curved at the top to reach in over the pubic bone. Could be worth investing in one.

● GET HER TO LIE ON HER STOMACH, hips raised on a pillow. Stimulate her as usual until she's aroused, then curl your fingers up behind her pubic bone about two inches inside her vagina. Now press behind her tummy button, making a 'come here' motion with your finger. The spot appears to respond to pressure – try rocking, massaging and making circling movements with your fingers (or the toy).

● USE THE OTHER HAND TO PRESS DOWN ON HER TUMMY just above the bikini line. If she says she feels like weeing, you're in the right area! (It's along the course of the urethra, which carries urine.)

● IF YOU CAN'T FEEL A LITTLE RAISED AREA and she's so bored, she's counting the threads on the bedspread, give up now. But what you may find, even if you don't find a G-spot, is that the whole area feels rather nice when touched in certain ways. Experiment with angles, fingers, toys and penises to get maximum benefit.

FIFTH PLACE
Sure Thing Sex Positions

Women who do orgasm through vaginal stimulation tend to have lots of clitoral or vulval stimulation beforehand (tons of good foreplay). So guys, it's generally a good idea to wait until she's massively aroused before moving into penetration, so you literally are just pushing her over the edge – in the nicest way possible. Up your chances of this happening by using G-spot/front wall-friendly positions. Any woman-on-top or rear-entry (best with her on her tummy) positions are good because you're aiming for shallow penetration angled toward her belly button. Other factors which can help give you the edge:

● **If she's on top,** get her to adjust her pelvis to ensure it rubs against the clitoris.

● **Get her to keep her legs together during intercourse** to create friction on the clitoris. (She should open her legs to allow you to penetrate, then close them once you're inside. You place your legs outside hers.)

● **If you shift your pelvis forward** during 'you on top' positions, you'll up the pressure and friction on the clitoris.

● **Keep thrusting slow and steady** – the sort the clitoris likes best! Give these twists on the traditional a spin.

Woman on top #1

He lies on his back, she sits on top of him (squatting or on her knees). She leans back, supporting her weight on her hands. He now makes a fist and places it on his lower abdomen so she can grind her clitoris against it. This ticks all the right boxes: it aims for the G-spot, adds clitoral stimulation, she controls the depth and pace – and he gets a nice view. (There is one con: the penis can slip out easily because it's at an odd angle.)

Woman on top #2

He lies on his back, she kneels astride him but facing away from him, not towards him. After he's penetrated, she should lean forward (towards his feet). He puts his hands on her hips to help lift her up and down, she holds onto the side of his thighs.

By facing away, you're directly hitting your target: the front wall.

Him behind

He stands behind and penetrates, then stands as upright as possible, hanging onto her hips with his hands. She keeps her legs straight and bottom lifted into his groin but leans down with her upper body, holding onto a bed or appropriate height surface for balance.

Man dominant

Make missionary so much better by getting her to pull her knees to her chest. Or try this one: she lies on her back on the bed, he kneels in front of her and lifts her legs under the knees so they're resting in the crook of his elbows. He lifts her up off the bed and by pulling up her hips, increases the pressure on the front wall.

SIXTH PLACE
Fabulously Fit Genitals

The stronger your vaginal muscles, the tighter you're able to contract your vagina around his penis. The tighter the grip, the higher the stimulation to the part of the clitoris which lies against the vaginal wall. (Remember, we just see the tip. Most of it is hidden.) Flexing the pubococcygeus (PC) muscle on a daily basis (see page 22) should keep your genitals nicely toned. Not only will it make you both a snugger fit, it could help you get in the mood. When females contract their 'sex muscle', they cause the walls of the vagina to contract which, in turn, causes an excretion of fluid. This is what happens during the excitement phase of sex, triggering your brain to think you're aroused now.

The most guaranteed way to give her an Orgasm

The answer is on the tip of his tongue. Given abysmal orgasm – during – intercourse statistics (twenty-five per cent on a good day), the odds increase rather dramatically when a tongue is substituted for a penis. A recent, reputable study found eighty-one per cent of women reach orgasm during oral sex. Forget grinding hips, it's all in the lips (and tongue and fingers and …). As with all the practical guides in sex books, this one provides helpful hints but don't think of it as the holy grail of cunnilingus. The only real expert on how and where they want to be stimulated is your partner. Use this as a starting point, then ask her what feels good and what doesn't:

● **DON'T DIVE STRAIGHT DOWN THERE** Lots of kissing, touching her breasts, stroking through her knickers, then gently using your hand to arouse her. Keep moving back up and away from the genitals to focus on her whole body: her breasts, her stomach, her thighs. The whole lot should feel touched and admired before you even think about starting. (Unless, of course, you're both highly aroused and in the mood for urgent, quick sex. In which case, a two-second snog might be all she needs!)

● **GET IN POSITION** They might look good in porn films but sixty-niners (both orally pleasuring each other simultaneously) aren't terribly effective. If someone's licking your bits, you aren't 100 per cent focused on what you're doing to theirs (and if you are, what's the point?). Getting her to sit on your face is also erotic but it stops you using your hands. Both are great places to start, but when you're ready to get serious about it, move into the following, even if it does sound boring: she lies on her back, legs apart but not massively so. Keeping her back flat rather than arched, get her to tilt her pelvis up toward your mouth. Popping a firm pillow under her bottom will help immeasurably.

● **THE TECHNIQUE** A good basic technique is to flatten your tongue and use the whole surface. Imagine you're licking an ice-cream which is about to drip everywhere! This stops it getting tired and it feels soft and gentle for her. You can

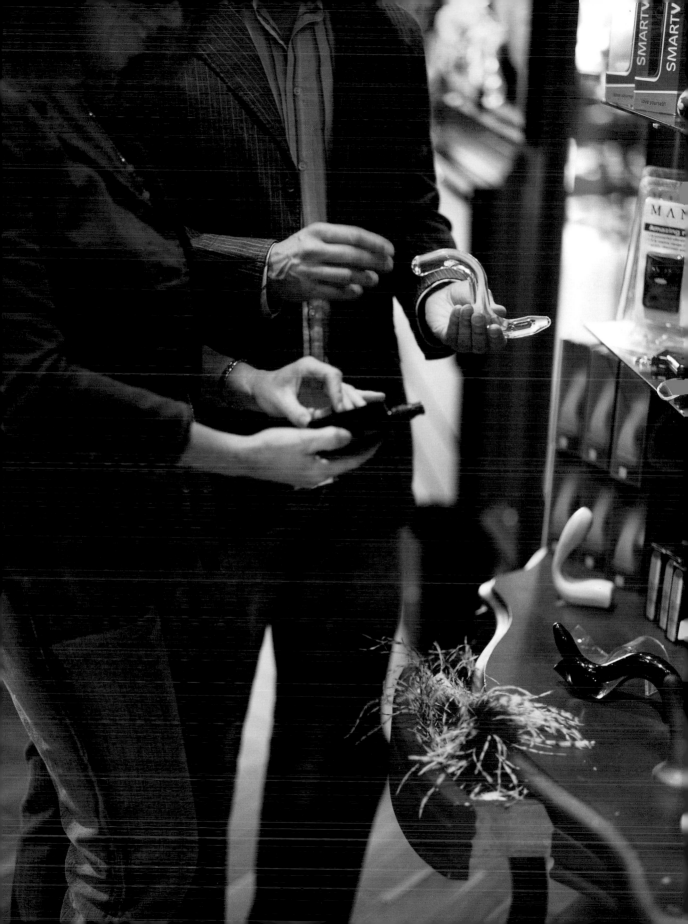

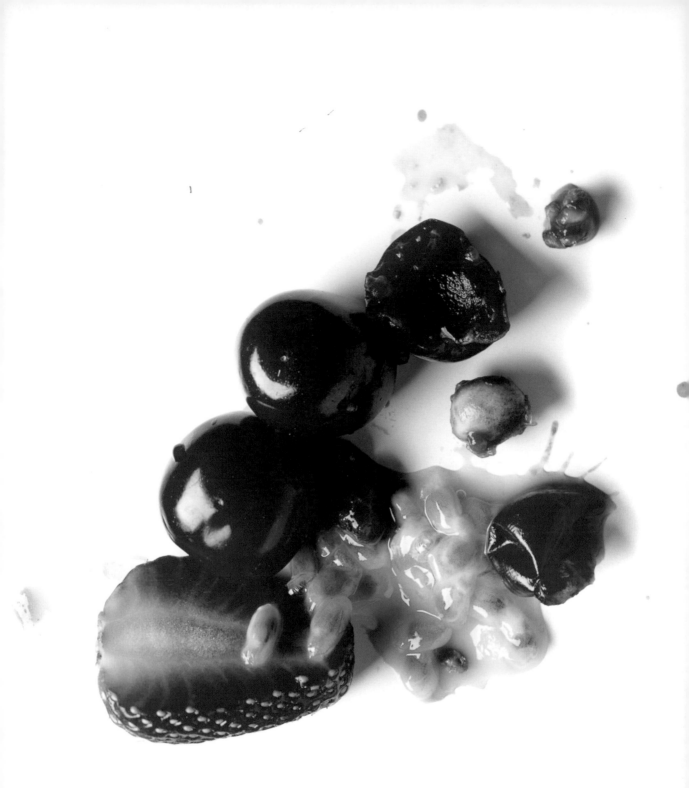

the female orgasm

'SOME WOMEN FIND IT EROTIC IF YOU TAKE A BREAK FROM ORAL AND COME BACK UP FOR A SEXY SNOG '

switch to different techniques – holding your tongue rigid and using the tip of your tongue only, for instance – for variety, but the 'flat tongue' is a good place to start. Go slow and be gentle (take a not-so-subtle tip from The Pointer Sisters – 'I want a lover with a slow hand, I want a lover with an easy touch.'). Gently wiggle your tongue around and over the clitoris or slide your whole tongue through the labia lips and then back again, skimming the clitoris as you go. The most important thing of all to remember: keep it consistent. Most women need consistent, steady rhythm to orgasm. If she seems to like what you're doing, stick with it rather than swap tongue techniques. (If your tongue is getting sore, consciously relax it rather than hold it stiff or move your head to move your tongue.)

● **USE YOUR HANDS** Play with her breasts with your spare hand, use both your hands to cup her buttocks and massage, insert a (lubricated) finger inside her vagina or anus, put a finger in her mouth so she can suck it and pretend she's returning the favour and sucking your penis. You're limited only by your imagination. Some women find it amazingly erotic if you take a break from giving her oral and come back up for a sexy snog. Others (Miranda from Sex and the City for one), find the whole concept of tasting 'themselves' repellent. Try it and see what reaction you get. If she kisses back passionately she finds the whole thing hot, if she turns her face so you hit her cheek possibly not. (If she runs straight for the bathroom sink shouting, 'Icky! Yuk!' start to worry. Unless you're happy having sex under the bedclothes with the lights out.)

● **DON'T STOP** Lots of women become very still and quiet just before orgasm, almost as though they're listening or waiting for it. If this happens, keep going. Keep going even if the roof falls in or your mother-in-law walks in the room. Keep going until she pushes you away (most clitorises get sensitive straight after), says 'Phew!' and reaches for water or generally gives a very clear sign that it's over. Thing is, female orgasms last longer than men's (you get five seconds, we get fifteen). You might think, 'There's no way she's still having one,' but she well might be. Hers last three times longer than yours. Tee hee! (Sorry to be smug, but come on, it takes us so long to get there, there's got to be a payoff!)

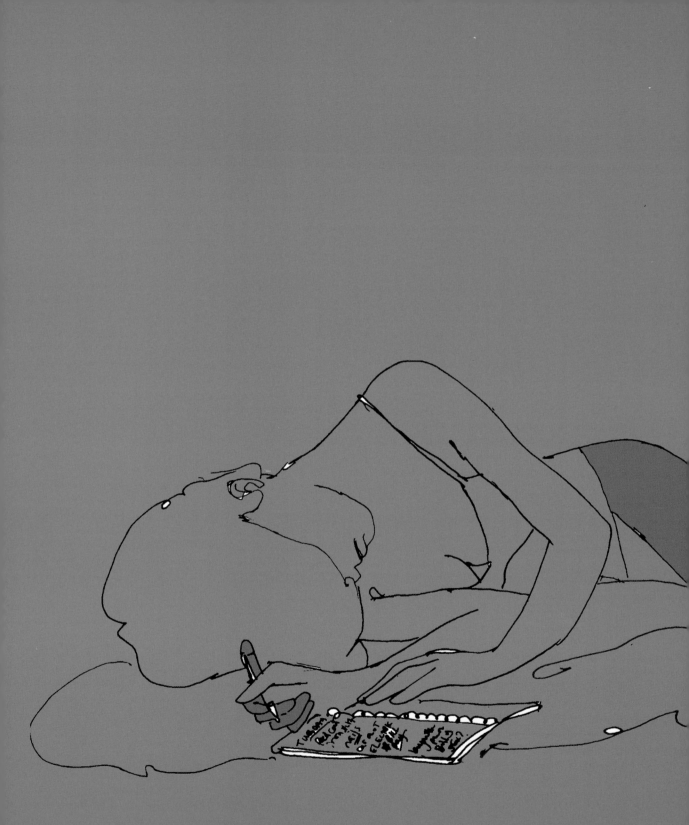

bored
by
monogamy

How to stop monogamy turning into monotony

ONOGAMY IS A WONDERFUL WAY for couples to experience the higher plane of love that exclusivity offers. And it can be quite a high. Sacrificing other sexual partners leads to a level of unity and intimacy that may not be achievable otherwise.

But if you're not careful, monogamy can turn into monotony. Your bedroom may have started out sounding like the final lap in the Grand Prix but it can easily start sounding like the clip-clop of a horse-drawn carriage.

If you're feeling that commitment is the death of sexual excitement you're wrong. It's actually the beginning. Because truly mind-blowing sex requires trust in addition to lust. Expressing the full range of your sexual desires requires someone that will support you physically and emotionally, and the most likely person to do that is the partner you're committed to.

bored by monogamy

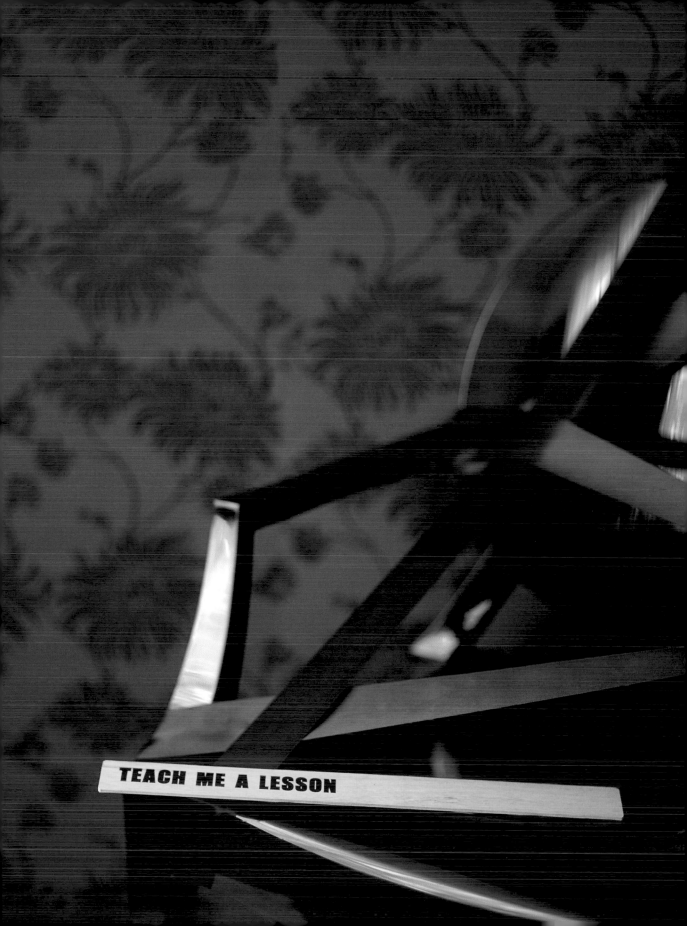

TEACH ME A LESSON

vanilla isn't the only
flavour to savour

HAVING SEX THE SAME WAY OVER AND OVER AGAIN is like going into an ice cream parlour with thirty-nine flavours and always ordering vanilla. There's nothing wrong with that, but maybe it's time to give vanilla a swerve. Imagine the delicious shock to your tastebuds when you sample the other thirty-eight flavours you haven't tried. This might translate to a specific activity (bondage, spanking), a special object (a piece of clothing, a sex toy, a bit of porn), a particular body part (feet, nipples, and necks) or just an idea, a fantasy or mindset (thinking of Becks and Posh spicing it up).

So what do you do when you're so familiar with your partner you know what they're going to do before they do? Just as achieving a greater love takes a lot of hard sacrifice, keeping that love takes a lot of hard play. That's right, play, not work. Because sex should never be work (unless you're getting paid for it, but really, that's another book).

ADDING SPICE ... BEFORE SOME OTHER CHEF BEATS YOU TO IT

There are all sorts of condiments to spice up your sex life – from a humble dash of salt and pepper to a huge helping of hair-straightening chilli sauce.

Sexual experimentation is a lot like cooking. It helps if you don't mind getting dirty. Or looking for the right tool. Or beating, whipping or pounding something into shape.

If you want to banish boredom, then author your own sexual cookbook. Take a pinch of this and a pinch of that and see how it tastes. If it works, keep it in the book. If it doesn't, stir in something that will. If it still doesn't taste right, throw it out.

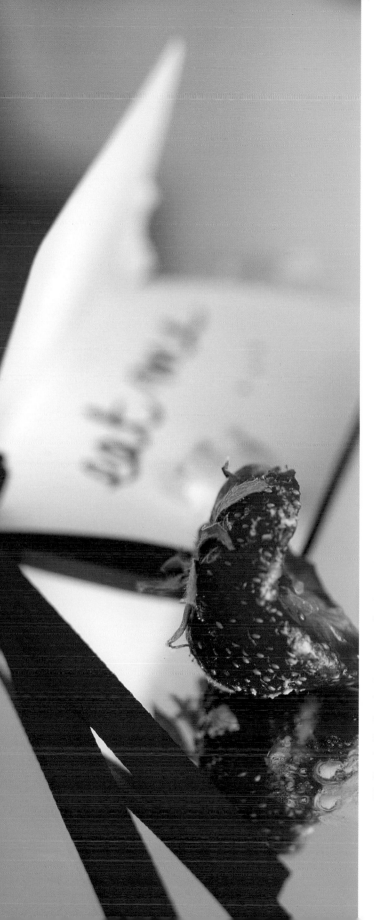

Sexual experimentation is a lot like cooking. It helps if you don't mind getting dirty

The best recipes always start with a good helping of Attitude. Bring a willingness to try things. A good chef is constantly licking the spoon, dipping his finger and stirring the pot. You should, too. Because the only way you're going to find out if you like something is to try it.

The most important thing about writing your sexual cookbook is your co-author. It's true that too many chefs in the kitchen spoil the meal, but like martinis, one's not enough and three's too many. Grab your fellow chef's hand and go about writing your book with the sense of wonder and fun you used to have as a kid, discovering new and forbidden mischief with your best friend.

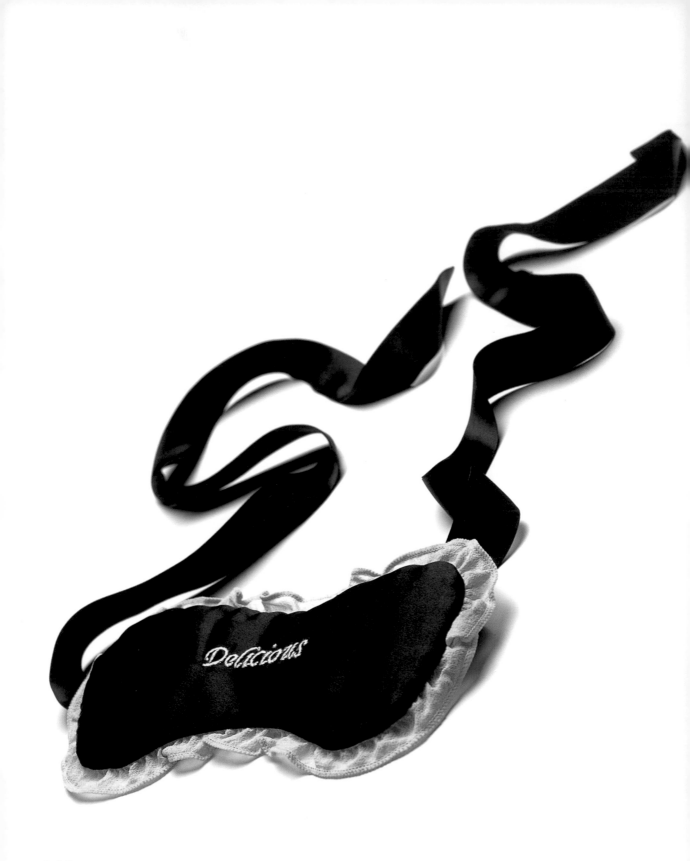

142
bored by monogamy

The *Sexual Inventory*

The first thing you both need to do is take your erotic temperature. Make a list. Remember what American sexologist Alfred Kinsey said, 'The only unnatural sex act is the one you can't perform.' Pick places, positions, fantasies, toys, roles, etc and list them on the left side of the paper. Then check your inner thermometer and circle the appropriate temperature. For example:

Spanking: *Cold*	*Cool*	*Lukewarm*	*Warm*	*Hot*
Blindfold: *Cold*	*Cool*	*Lukewarm*	*Warm*	*Hot*
Standing: *Cold*	*Cool*	*Lukewarm*	*Warm*	*Hot*
Kitchen: *Cold*	*Cool*	*Lukewarm*	*Warm*	*Hot*

DONE? CONGRATULATIONS! Now you've got a list of things you're dying to try, wanting to try, trying to try and no-way-you're-going to try. Take each other's lists and compare them. Have a go at the things you've both circled as lukewarm-to-hot. You might bet you'll know your partner's answers but trust me, you're in for a couple of surprises. Every time we did a sexual inventory on *The Sex Inspectors* the couples were stunned at the desires their partners voiced. Take Nick and Sarah, for example. Nick was the adventurous one; Sarah the shy one. Or so he thought. I remember Nick looking at the circled lists, turning to Sarah and saying, 'I'll be damned. Not in a million years did I think you'd go for that.' Sarah blushed, looked at the ground and said, 'Because you never asked, darling.'

bored by monogamy

space matters

ADDING A LITTLE PIZAZZ TO YOUR LOVE LIFE might just be a matter of changing locations. Depending on what you have in mind – and local ordinances – that may entail planning a weekend in Amsterdam or simply moving things to the lounge or the kitchen.

Create a place that won't distract, judge or inhibit. If your bedroom's your only option then use your imagination to turn it from a place you snore in to a place you moan in. For example: every second Tuesday, from eight to midnight, the bedroom becomes a bubble. On the appointed day and at the appointed hour, you step through the bubble into a fantasyland. You leave behind your everyday selves and for the next few hours become The Rock Star and His Groupie or The Mistress and the Stable Boy.

EXPLORING SPACE

How do you create or discover a special place for sex?

● **MOVE IT AROUND** It doesn't take much to make a room look and feel different. Cover the furniture with sheets. Or move everything to one side, lay a futon in the middle and circle it with candles to create a kind of sexual altar.

● **STEAM IT UP** Messy play with food or other substances is so much more convenient in the shower, where you can steam and stream the mess away.

● **TAKE A HIKE** Put a little angle in your tangle by using the stairs. If they aren't carpeted, get some subtle padding. If you really want to get twisted, try a winding staircase.

● **TAKE A BITE** Apples, bananas and kumquats, oh my! The kitchen is the logical place for 'food sex', what with all the counter tops, work surfaces and utensils.

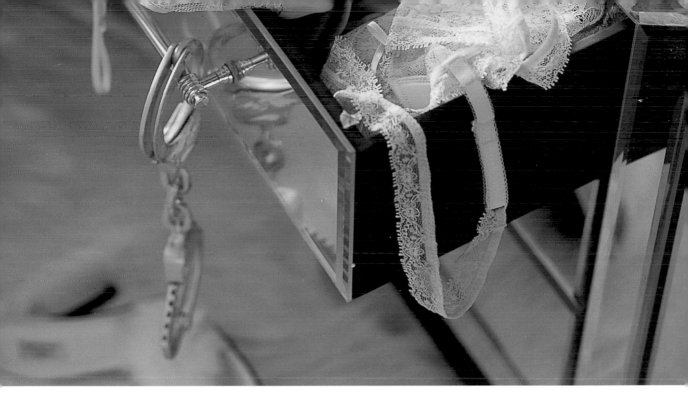

If your loved one can't see your facial expressions, it'll leave them with a tingling curiosity

PUBLIC SEX, PRIVATE CELL

Sex in a park or in a cinema or behind the town hall may turn you on, but that busload of nuns who caught your matinee act did not give their consent to see what they saw. Public sex may be an aphrodisiac but it's also grounds for arrest. Trust me, that Prisoner/Warden thing is much better as a fantasy than a reality.

THE BLIND LEADING THE BLIND

Blindfolds serve as the most basic sort of bondage. They're a great way to experience the exhilaration of sensory deprivation. By subtracting one sense, blindfolds require the other four to work harder. Without vision, two hands can feel like four or six. You're not sure where the next touch or probe is going to come from. Sensations are heightened. Plus, you can conjure up whoever you'd like to star in the show. Add a gag and it means that you have to communicate exclusively through touch and body responses. Very intense.

Checklist

Of course, you don't want to be too obvious, but remember, luck favours the prepared. If you're smooth enough, the champagne seems to appear from nowhere – already chilled. And the padded handcuffs appear from nowhere – already warmed.

CONSIDER DOING SOME BASIC PREP WORK:

● MOMENT OF MAD PASSION If you think you might throw your love onto the dining table in a moment of mad passion, you might weight test the platform once or twice and reinforce as required. Nothing shatters the mood like collapsing furniture – or picking splinters out of each other's bums.

● HAVE CONDOMS AND LUBE READY at various stations, always within easy reach.

● IF YOU INTEND TO PLAY with something like handcuffs, it's not a bad idea to have several handcuff keys stashed at strategic places around the house (like, right next to the lube).

● MINIMIZE POTENTIAL INTERRUPTIONS Clear your schedule. Turn the phones off. Don't order take-away for delivery (unless the delivery boy is part of the fantasy). Don't answer the door unless it's the local fire brigade.

● PLAN FOR THE AFTERGLOW (something besides rolling over and going to sleep). Some activities can be rather intense and your partner can feel a little silly or panicky afterwards. Bring the mood down slowly and gently. Have a cuddle, a talk, a snack. And always tip the delivery boy.

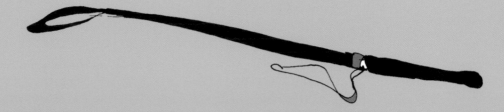

role play and fantasy

THE HUMAN MIND IS AN AMAZING THING. It can transform one or both of you into someone else. Remember the games you used to play as a kid? Well, you can play them as adults, only with an added zing. You can play The Prisoner and the Camp Guard, The Gladiator and the Slave Girl, or The Hunter and the Lonely Shepherdess. The roles, costuming and staging can be complex or simple … depending on your ability to suspend disbelief. Use the opportunity to step outside yourself, to be someone you're usually not but have always wanted to be. Tracey and John, a lovely couple we worked with in *The Sex Inspectors*, wanted to do more role-play but didn't know how. John was a rather shy, timid fellow while Tracey was a confident, take-charge mum who pretty much ran the house. They wanted to reverse roles in bed. Tracey wanted to be bossed around, while John wanted to feel what it was like to be in complete control. We suggested something that shocked them: film it.

They asked me exactly what you're probably asking yourself right now – why? Why not do it without a video camera? Because making the video forces you to put structure around the role-playing. It's fine to say that one of you wants to play the cigarette while the other plays the ashtray, but where do you start? What kind of cigarette? What colour ashtray? Is the cigarette already lit or will somebody light it? By being the scriptwriter, producer, director, even the lighting technician, you'll end up with a much more powerful experience of your fantasies.

Use the opportunity to step outside yourself, to be someone you're usually not

POWER EXCHANGE

All couples are inherently unequal. One partner always has more money, beauty, charm, athleticism, energy or power at any given time. The idea of power exchange is to recognize – even celebrate – this inequality. It can express the natural structure of your relationship, or occasionally allow both of you to switch roles, perhaps allowing the less assertive or less dominant partner to rule. If the man is the head of the house and chief decision-maker, perhaps he could spend an evening as The Loin-clothed Slave Boy serving the every whim of his Nile Princess. Likewise, if the woman is the primary household manager and instigator, perhaps she can take a break and simply follow the instructions of her Lord. Submission and domination can be traded and played with like cards.

Serving another human can be very educational. To put another's pleasure first you may discover much about yourself and much about your partner.

BONDAGE

Light restraint can be exciting in several ways. Just the physical sensation of being confined can be erotic. Some people like the way bonds feel on the wrists or ankles, or how the positions show off muscle tone. For some, getting tied up gives them permission to enjoy what they otherwise wouldn't allow: 'What could I do? I was tied up … I had no choice but to lie back and have a good time.'

Almost any sexual position has bondage possibilities, and nearly any bondage configuration has sexual possibilities. Spread-eagle (hands and feet each tied to the four corners of the bed) is very common and reasonably comfortable, but you might also try binding arms together and feet together.

To begin, use soft bindings that spread pressure out, not cord or rope that cuts into flesh. If you really want to, you can spend a fortune on specially made restraints, cuffs and harnesses from sex shops. Whether they're homemade or shop-bought, check bonds often to make sure there aren't any cuts, bruises or loss of circulation. Release at the first sign of numbness or tingling.

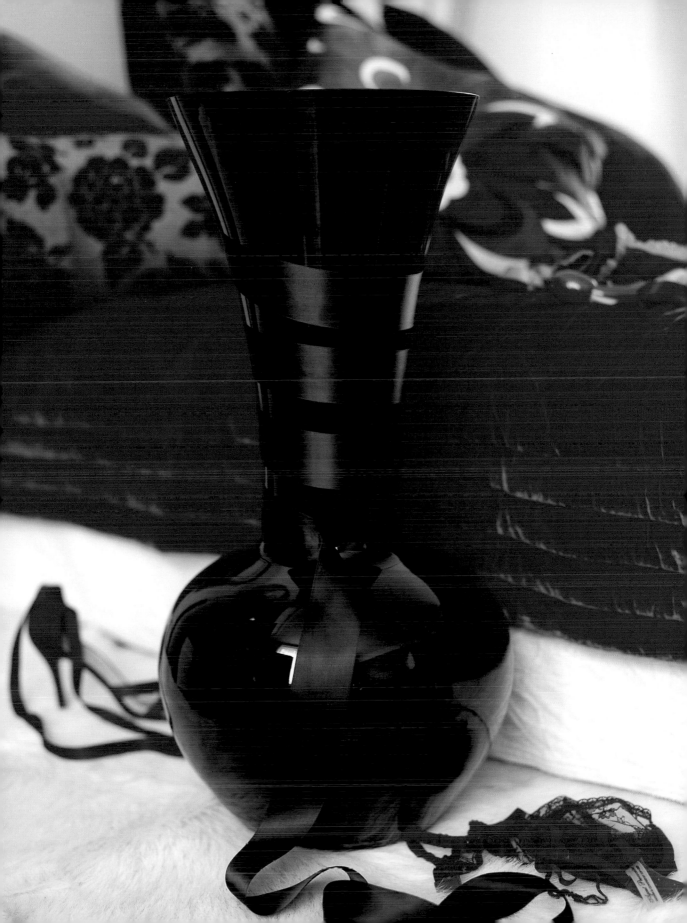

'IF YOU'RE FEELING THAT COMMITMENT IS THE DEATH OF SEXUAL EXCITEMENT, YOU'RE WRONG. IT'S THE BEGINNING '

'NO, STOP, DON'T. NO, DON'T STOP'

'Consensual non-consensuality' may sound like a contradiction in terms but it's an important principle in sex play. It's simply the voluntary surrender of your right to say 'no'. It means you've agreed to be kidnapped and forced to do whatever your captor says, or you've agreed to be the slave to an all-commanding master who must be obeyed. It is creating the illusion that you have no choice.

Creating no-choice situations can only be done safely by granting consent, which in turn requires trust. Would you really let someone you can't depend on tie you to the tracks of an oncoming train for a rescue fantasy? Your motto should be 'No Trust, No Truss'. Relinquishing power magnifies the impact of a fantasy so carefully negotiate lines you don't want crossed, lest psychological damage be done.

Spared from change

ANY SUDDEN CHANGE IN SEXUAL ROUTINE CAN OFTEN BE TAKEN AS A SIGN YOU'RE CHEATING ON YOUR LOVER. AFTER ALL, YOUR PARTNER MIGHT BE THINKING, 'I SURE AS HELL DIDN'T TEACH HIM THAT! WHO DID?!' MAKE SURE YOU COMMUNICATE WITH YOUR PARTNER – SPECIFICALLY TO LET THEM KNOW WHERE YOU LEARNT IT, E.G. THIS BOOK – THAT YOU WANT TO RESUSCITATE THE RELATIONSHIP, NOT END IT.

fun with food

SOMETIMES LOVE CAN BE MESSY. Adding food to sex works on so many levels. Even before we were told, 'Don't play with yourself!' we were told, 'Don't play with your food!' It's rebellious, childish, playful. And delicious.

Food has an endless variety of textures, temperatures, flavours, shapes and sizes to play with. Beyond the basic cucumber, you   are limited only by your tastes and imagination. Well, that and the expiration dates.

Some tips...

Yogurt can create sensuous goo for two bodies to slide together. Champagne sipped from the foreskin presents a decadent type of (ahem) stemware. Chilled fruit can cause quite a sensation when inserted into various orifices and withdrawn with a warm tongue. Drip ice over breasts, or smother in ice cream to then lick off! Over the page there are some more tips to make sure Food Sex doesn't give you indigestion:

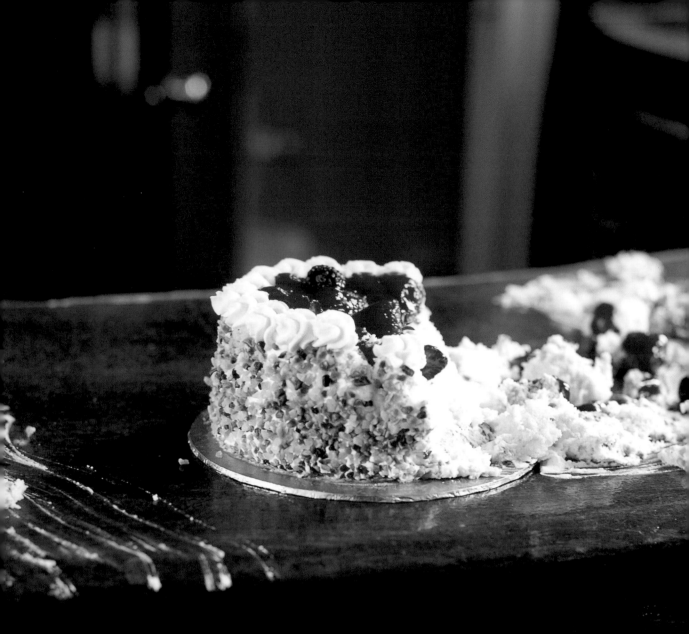

The setting

YOUR KITCHEN FLOOR. *He sits with his back to the wall.* YOU CAN **BLINDFOLD** HIM BUT IT'S MORE *powerful* IF HE SIMPLY *closes his eyes* AND **TRUSTS** YOU.

The shopping list

FOOD OF EVERY TEXTURE, SMELL AND TASTE IMAGINABLE: SOFT, HARD, CHEWY, *salty*, SWEET, BITTER. BEST BETS: *maraschino cherries*, JELLY, PEPPERS, STRAWBERRIES, *curly pasta (cooked, don't be cruel)*, GRAPES (SEEDLESS, DON'T BE MEAN), *eggs(boiled, don't be hateful)*, AND OLIVES (PITTED, DON'T BE HEARTLESS).

The deed

With his eyes closed, feed him a piece of each FOOD. But don't just feed him, *tease* him. Take a grape and tap it from the bridge of his nose to his lips before plopping it in his mouth. Let the SYRUP RUN ON HIS CHIN before feeding him a spoonful of maraschino cherries. Encourage him to *play* with the food by *licking his lips,* sticking out his tongue, savouring the flavours. Two rules for him: EYES SHUT AND NO HANDS. He's not allowed to touch you. The secret to making it *sexy* is to deprive him of some senses (touch and sight), enhancing the others *(smell and taste).* The UNPREDICTABILITY of what you'll do next also creates a thrilling anticipation. You won't believe how sexy it is to hold a plastic bottle of HONEY, ask that he stick his TONGUE out and watch the honey *ooze* out and pool in his tongue. Make sure you wash down the food with different liquids – *milk, juice, water.* For added effect, drink some WINE, hold it in your mouth and SQUIRT it into his. Then get a mop and a bucket. Not for HIM! For everything around him.

forget the roses
send me the thorns

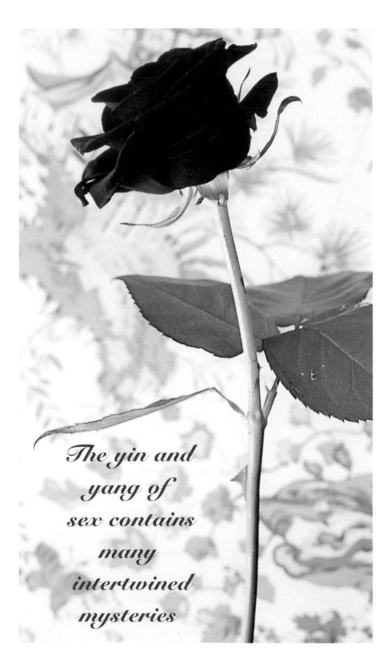

The yin and yang of sex contains many intertwined mysteries

ON *THE SEX INSPECTORS,* WE DISCOVERED a surprising number of couples that enjoyed a bit of light pain. Spanking can make even the stiffest upper lip quiver with delight. 'Didn't take out the rubbish when I asked?' Spank. 'Bad boy!'

The yin and yang of sex contains many intertwined mysteries, not the least of which is the paradox between pain and pleasure. 'Pain' can mean many different things to different people, but you do need to be very clear about what level is pleasurable to you. Physically, pain releases a chemical rush of endorphins that some people enjoy. From a psychological point of view, it gets your attention and focuses you on the moment.

Administering pain comes in all sorts of forms. There is 'percussion', which is basically light spanking. Tickling is another form. Always be careful. I have seen more problems between couples arise over tickling that got out of hand (issues of mixed messages and childhood trauma) than what many would consider more 'serious' pain.

Checklist

If you're a fan of flagellation then by all means, ask your partner to bend you over their knee for a spot of spanking. But as with fantasy or role-play, it pays to be prepared:

● ANY SPANKING (even with an open hand) can cause bruises or raise welts. Be careful and be gentle.

● PADDLES AND FLOGGERS with a wide surface tend to do less damage to the skin. Stick to items that give a 'thudding' rather than 'stinging' sensation. Avoid narrow-ended whips or riding crops unless they are just for show when acting out a fantasy (they can really sting).

● WHEN TRYING OUT A NEW ACTIVITY do a little role reversal first. If someone wants you to spank them, have them give you one or two spanks to see precisely what they have in mind. Experiencing what they want gives you the opportunity to adjust the intensity. Besides, taking a little of what you're dishing out isn't such a bad idea.

● PRACTISE MAKES PERFECT Having a good aim and finding the right level of strength is important. The most erotic part of the body for this activity is the lower part of the buttocks, but don't hit exactly the same spot over and over as you could cause cuts or lacerations.

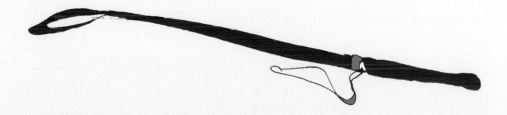

SAFETY FIRST

Sometimes, as we explore a sexual frontier, we confront very powerful forces. Those should be treated with respect and a certain amount of preparation. There are three types of possible mishap: **a physical problem (injury, burn, bruise, etc), an environmental problem (fire, power outage, etc) or an emotional problem (panic attack, depression, etc).**

THE BEST WAY TO MITIGATE ANY EMERGENCY IS TO PREVENT IT IN THE FIRST PLACE.

● KNOW YOUR PARTNER. Are there any health problems? Any chronic conditions? Any psychological triggers?

● COMMUNICATE WITH YOUR PARTNER. Look for any signs of anxiety or panic. Consider using a communications device such as a 'safeword' (explained below).

● SPEND A MOMENT OR TWO and ask yourself, 'What could possibly go wrong with my plans?' Then plan for each contingency.

● WATCH SOURCES OF IGNITION LIKE CANDLES AND HEATERS. Plan ahead so they won't become a problem later when your mind is on other sources of ignition.

● IF YOU ARE PLAYING WITH BONDAGE OR RESTRAINT, how will you release the restraints in an emergency? Have safety scissors ready to cut bindings. Use the blunt-ended kind used in hospitals.

● FOR ROPE BONDAGE, study knot tying (a Boy Scout manual is excellent for this purpose). You don't need to memorize the whole book, just find a few knots you can practise, become comfortable with and know their characteristics. You want to avoid slip-knots (which tighten as pull is applied) and learn quick release knots (which can be untied in just one or two movements).

● CHECK WITH MARITIME OR SAILING SUPPLY HOUSES. There are many quick-release systems for sailboat rigging and lines that are practical for home use.

● DEPENDING ON YOUR LEVEL OF PLAY, consider having the following on your speed dial: emergency services, your doctor, a trusted and non-judgemental friend, a lawyer or a locksmith.

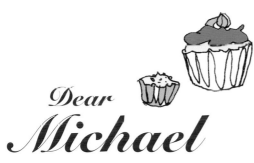

Dear *Michael*

MY GIRLFRIEND AND I HAVE TRIED TO HAVE
ANAL SEX A COUPLE OF TIMES BUT SHE
SAYS IT HURTS TOO MUCH. WHAT ARE WE
DOING WRONG?

Pain during intercourse is a signal that
something is wrong. It's not unusual to
feel pain, even when you are gentle.
There are, however, some basic steps to
easier anal sex. The first thing is lots of
lubrication. Lubricate your finger and get
familiar with the contours of her outer
sphincter and SLOWLY move in. Every
time she says it feels like it might hurt
back off a little. Once she gets used to
your fingers, go to a sex shop and buy
three dildos: small, medium and YOU.
First, slowly insert the small, well-lubricated dildo. The outer and inner ring of the
sphincter will lighten. The outer ring is
controlled voluntarily but the inner ring is
involuntary. As her body recognizes that
the foreign object is not going to hurt it,
it'll loosen up on its own. Push the toy in
a little further and go through the same
process. Next, graduate to the medium-
sized toy and then to your size. Now
she's ready for the real thing. Enter her
using the same process: Push, stop, relax.
Push, stop, relax. It's really important that
you see this as a process and not an
event.

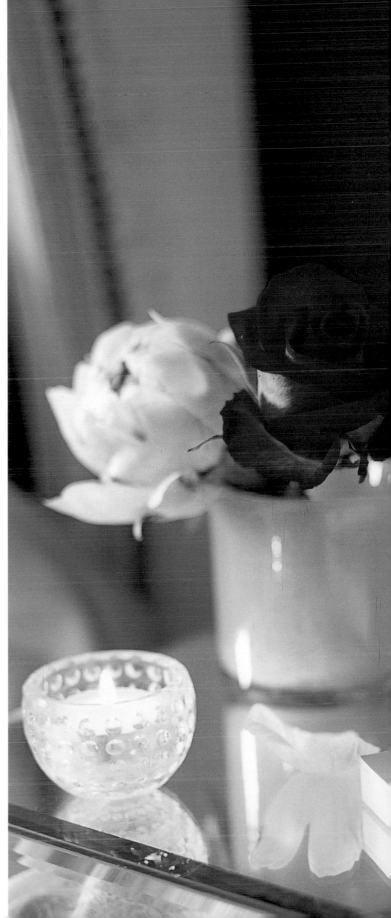

CHOOSE A SAFEWORD

Safewords are a device; a code that instantly suspends the action. Think of it as pulling the emergency brake cord on a trolley or inventing a secret signal to cut short a boring cocktail party. 'Safewords' are in code because they can break the action without breaking the mood. They also allow action to continue once the requisite strap is adjusted, the muscle cramp is massaged away or the offending object is removed from the violated orifice.

Don't pick safewords like 'No' or 'Stop' because you may want to shout them in the thrill of a struggle. Choose words that connote the end of something. Like 'Lease' (breaking a lease) or 'Caesar' (cease and desist).

Safewords can be a simple on/off switch or a much more complex, multi-level system, such as 'Red' ('Please stop, I have reason to fear injury'), 'Yellow' ('I can continue if you proceed with caution') and 'Green' ('Press the booster rocket, baby, I'm headed for the moon!').

EVERYDAY ITEMS AS SEX TOYS

Nearly everything has the potential to be a sex toy.

● **SILK NECKTIES** They're strong but can't really cut into ankles or wrists. Ladies, just don't grab his precious Eton stripe tie. At that point the torture moves to an entirely different level.

● **CLING FILM** An excellent bondage media because with the right holes in the right places you can wrap your lover like a leftover. This is often called 'mummification'. Just make sure you do it from the neck down! We want the mummy in a bed, not a coffin.

● **DUCT TAPE** is popular for bondage art. It is strong and wide enough to avoid cutting off circulation. Be careful about putting it on a hairy man, though. You want him screaming your name, not bloody murder. Try putting a layer of cling film under the tape before binding.

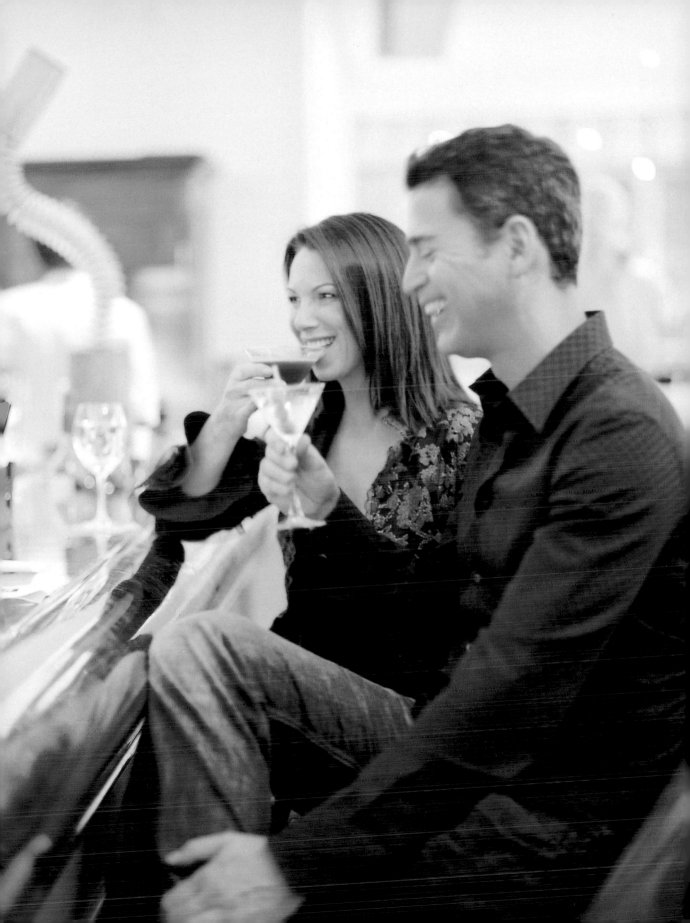

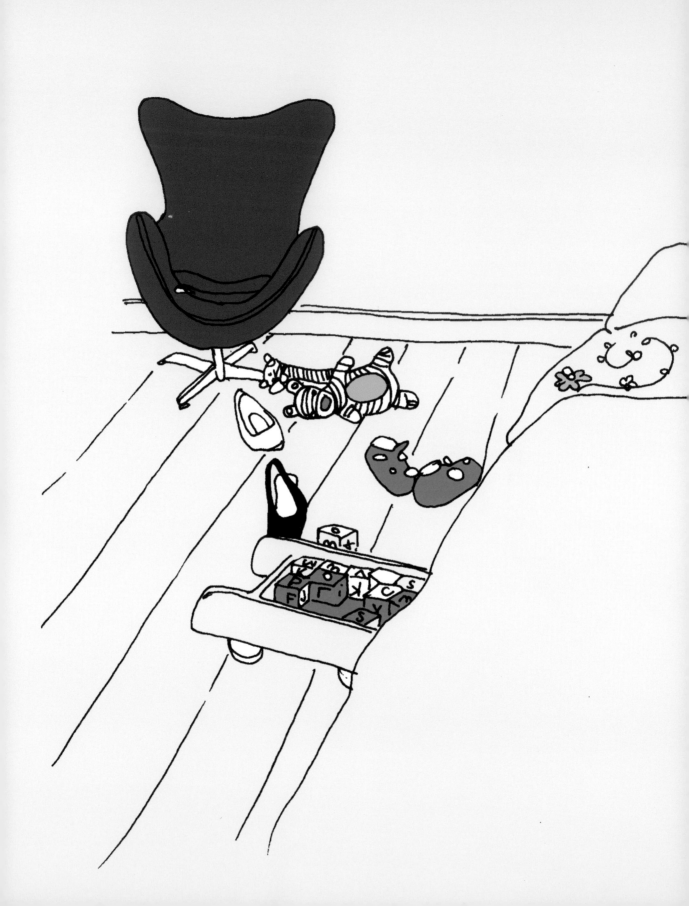

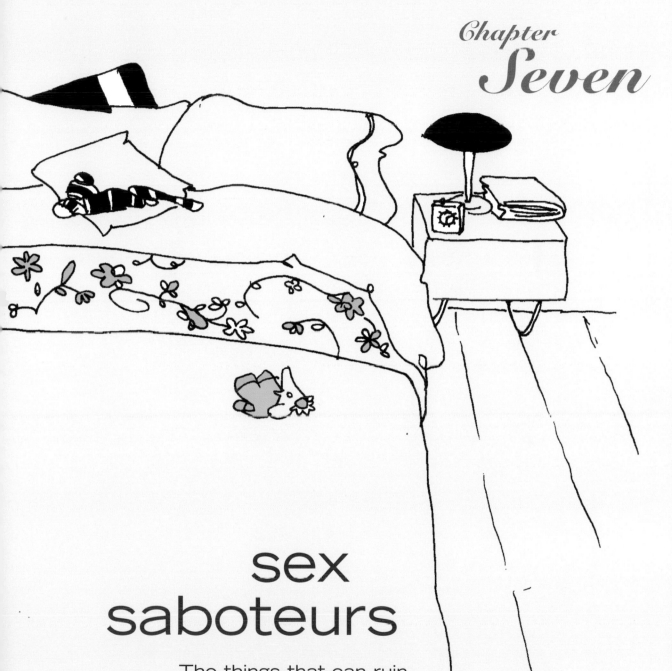

sex saboteurs

The things that can ruin
your sex life and how to
overcome them

WHODUNIT? WHO KILLED YOUR SEX LIFE? The kids? Drugs? Alcohol? A porn addiction? From serious conditions like asthma to smelly conditions like halitosis, there are lots of factors that can sabotage your sex life.

Fortunately, plenty of aerial reconnaissance has been done on these sex saboteurs and we know how to neutralize them. Knowledge is power and you can use it to resuscitate your love life. Sometimes, knowing a small fact can make all the difference in the world. For example, a simple change in position can allow asthmatics to have sex. Sometimes knowing you're not alone can give you hope. For example, sixty-six per cent of women report low libidos after giving birth. And sometimes, knowing what not to do is more helpful than knowing what to do. For example, don't drink that fourth pint if you want to perform in bed.

Knowledge will take you far. But not nearly as far as love, patience and kindness. Have some compassion for yourself and your partner. Your sex life didn't go south overnight; it won't go north in the same time frame either. Let's take a look at the most common things that can drive a stake through the heart of your sex life and how we can fix it.

'66% OF WOMEN REPORT HAVING LOW LIBIDOS AFTER GIVING BIRTH...'

Think you're alone? Think again...

A WOMAN'S LIBIDO is usually very low for up to a year after childbirth, simply due to exhaustion.

TWO THIRDS OF WOMEN report the frequency of sex decreases after their children are born.

TEN PERCENT OF COUPLES don't have sex for a full year after their child arrives.

BY A CHILD'S FIRST BIRTHDAY, couples have sex an average of once a week

FROM RAISING HELL TO RAISING KIDS

Let's be blunt: Nothing kills a sex life faster than kids. If orgasms were financial institutions, giving birth is the equivalent of a stock market crash. Every market indicator goes south – your libido, your sense of adventure, your sensual attraction to your partner. Like any investment that lost its value, you have to be patient to gain it back. And patience begins by first understanding the nature of the problem.

It isn't easy, going from a hell-raising, barn-burning 'must-have' sex life to a yawn inducing, eye-rolling, 'must-you?' love trap. But kids will do that. Yes, they're the apple of your eye. Yes, they've given you a new meaning, a new purpose to life. But they've also sapped your sexual energy. Now, instead of dropping your drawers at the door, you're closing the door on your drawers.

What happened? And, more importantly, how can you make it better? First, you need to know it's completely normal to feel a drop in desire after the birth of a baby. Low libido is pretty much the rule for women who've given birth. Some scientists believe it's nature's way of assuring healthier families (no libido means no sex, which spaces out the kids more, giving mothers a break).

And don't forget, you didn't just run off to the pound and adopt a

Now, instead of dropping your drawers at the door, you're closing the door on your drawers

puppy. Your body went through an internal hurricane. Glands packing gale-force winds caused hormonal hailstorms, battering you from elation to depression like a canoe in a squall. Your brain sent emergency broadcast signals to every part of your body, ordering supplies and barking out evacuation routes. What made you hungry one minute made you nauseous the next. And to top it all off, the only good news (your breasts are bigger!) is offset by the bad (they're so tender and swollen you don't want anybody touching them).

Well, no wonder you don't want to have sex! Who would? Men have no idea what women go through when they give birth. Oh, sure, we're in the delivery room. But we'll never really know what it feels like. That's why, when obstetricians give the green light to sex four to six weeks after delivery (the typical waiting time) men rub their hands in glee while women rub their knees with glue.

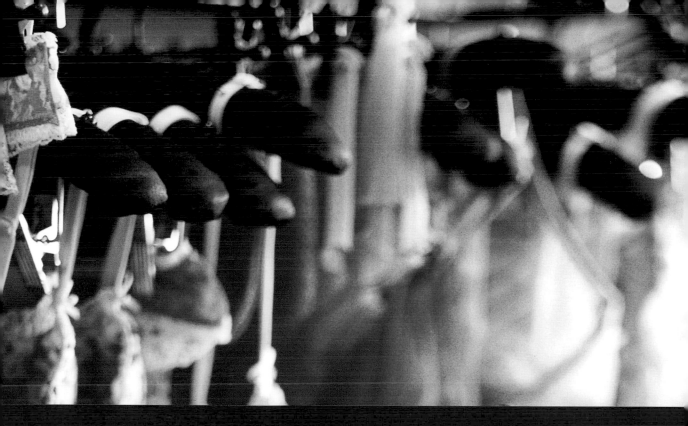

YOU WANT IT. SHE DOESN'T. HERE'S WHY

● **SORENESS** Lacerations or stitches after childbirth make sex painful.

● **RECOVERY FROM SURGERY** Any surgery takes time to recover from. But the trauma is deeper when you have a caesarean section (pulling the baby out through a cut in the stomach and uterus rather than being pushed out of the vagina).

● **ANAEMIA** A deficiency in healthy red blood cells, the main transporter of oxygen, often develops in new mothers, saddling them with fatigue, dizziness and difficulty in concentrating.

● **A NEW ROLE FOR THE BREASTS** Once you whip out a breast in the middle of a grocery store to feed a baby, you start thinking of them as bottles, not jugs. What was once strictly a fun factor becomes a food factory, too, making some women ambivalent about the sexiness of their breasts.

● **STRETCH MARKS** They happen when a body part, oh say, the one carrying the baby, grows faster than the skin can cover it. Though the red or purplish wavy lines become fine, white and silvery over time, nothing takes them away. And that can make a woman feel she's not attractive enough to have sex.

endless days/sleepless nights

ONCE THE BABY'S BORN, the hurricane moves out of your body and into the house. Now you've got to take care of someone who wants what it wants when it wants it, waking you up in the middle of the night whining and crying if it doesn't get its way. But enough about your husband.

Seriously, the relentless needs of a child shift your priorities the way pregnancy shifted your body. You used to stay up all night with your partner. Now you're up all night with the baby. And it doesn't get much easier when they grow up. From cooling toddler temper tantrums to getting pre-schoolers to bed, to driving kids to school, you're no longer a sexual being. You're a maid, a chauffeur, a cook, a nurse, a teacher, a disciplinarian, a coach, and a milk-dispenser. With their new, all-consuming role, many women say they just don't 'need' men anymore. They're having all their physical needs satisfied – cuddling, touching, nurturing. It's not unusual for women to literally cringe when their husbands touch them in a way they know leads to sex. I remember Tracey and John, a couple we helped in *The Sex Inspectors*. Tracey asked, 'If I don't want to have sex, does that mean I've gone off him?' She wrongly interpreted her lack of sexual desire as a loss of love for her boyfriend. It wasn't that she'd gone off him; it was that she'd gone from lover to mum and wasn't ready to balance both roles yet.

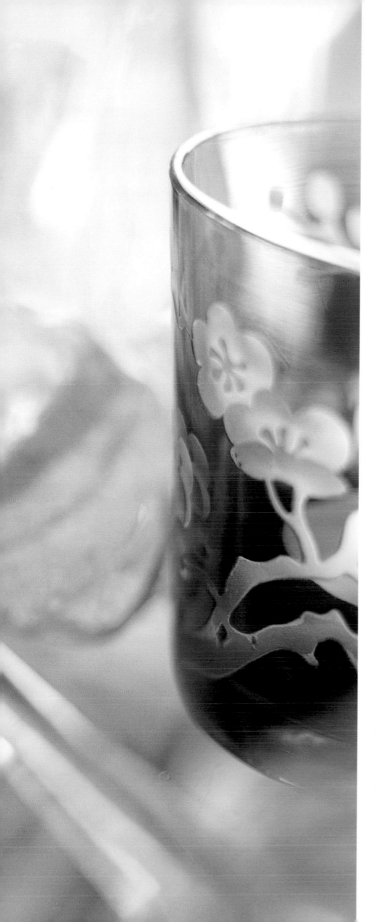

How hormones turn her moans into groans

● BREAST-FEEDING The ovaries make a small amount of testosterone, a key ingredient to charging up libidos, but breast-feeding suppresses ovarian production of this vital hormone, sucking the life out of her libido.

● POSTPARTUM DEPRESSION Almost a third of all mothers experience this debilitating disorder. Crying spells, anxiety attacks, and sleeplessness (even when the baby's asleep) make sex impossible.

● PROLACTIN This hormone stimulates milk production, which suppresses oestrogen, drying out the entire region below the belt and making sex painful.

Now that we've defined the problem, let's look at the four main solutions:

GIVE YOURSELF A BREAK!

Women's Cues Pretend your best friend is going through everything you just read. What would you tell her? 'Quit whining? Let him have his way and get it over with'? Please. Be as kind and compassionate to yourself as you would be to her. Time may be a lousy beautician but it's a great healer. You'll get your groove back as long as you let time work its magic.

Men's Clues Sorry, mate. Time to fly solo. Yes, you'll have to take your wallet out and show people a picture of your hand instead of your wife, but it's only temporary. And do it when she's not around (the masturbating, not the wallet-showing) otherwise you'll just add to the guilt she already feels about her low libido.

Every fire starts with a spark. Make her feel like she's the love of your life, not just the mother of your kids

GIVE YOURSELF A BRAKE!

Women's Cues Put the brakes on the mummy car every once in a while. Get out, stretch and hitch a ride to Lover's Lane. Your partner will be more than glad to pick you up. Set boundaries for yourself. Not every dish has to be washed, not every shirt has to be ironed, not every room has to be vacuumed. Place yourself higher on your 'To Do' list. Pamper yourself: facials, manicures, pedicures. How will you find the time? Delegate, enlist, enroll. You've got family and friends that'll help if you ask and babysitters that'll help if you pay.

Men's Clues She's not a one-woman show. Share the stage. Help out. Take the kids out to the park without her. YOU arrange for the babysitter. Take turns putting the kids to bed. And most importantly, make friends with the mop. Surveys show UK women do three-quarters of the housework, spending almost nineteen hours a week on household chores compared to six hours for the average man. If you want more sex, do more housework.

TAKE RESPONSIBILITY FOR YOUR OWN SENSUALITY

Women's Cues Don't wait for the mood to strike; strike into the mood. How? The same way you get yourself to do anything you don't feel like doing – work up to it. How do you get to the gym when you feel like napping? Play high-energy music, sing loudly and watch your energy creep back. How do you eat when you're not hungry? Take a small bite of something delicious and feel your appetite return. How do you make love when you're not up for it? Start with light kissing in sensitive areas and feel your libido warm up. For more ideas, see Tracey's chapter on low libidos.

Men's Clues Forget the 'wham, bam, thank you ma'am' school of foreplay. Those days are gone. Try 'beforeplay.' Spritz a little cologne and walk by her so she gets a whiff as you walk by. Sneak up from behind, cover her eyes, whisper something sexy in her ear, and walk away. Every fire starts with a spark and it's your job to rub some sticks together. Make her feel like she's the love of your life, not just the mother of your kids.

MAKE LOVE FOR THE KIDS NOT JUST TO GET THE KIDS

Women's Cues If your world revolves around the kids, then it's even more important that you have a good sex life. Sexually satisfied parents are more affectionate, have more fun and settle their differences respectfully, modelling positive behaviour for their children. Nick and Katie, a couple we helped on *The Sex Inspectors*, couldn't believe the impact their improved sex life had on their five year old and three year old. 'They're fighting less and hugging more,' said Katie. 'I guess it's true – "happy families, happy children."'

Men's Clues Be demonstratively affectionate in front of the kids. Happier kids decrease 'mummy stress', leaving her more energy for you. Besides, the more you make her feel loved during the day the more she'll make love to you at night. And no 'foreploy'. You know, misrepresenting your affections as a way of getting sex. Only no-agenda cuddles and kisses allowed.

must-haves for

Parents

A LOCK ON THE BEDROOM DOOR, A PORTABLE RADIO THAT CAN BE MOVED CLOSE TO THE DOOR, A BEDROOM PHONE THAT DISCONNECTS EASILY, A LOCKABLE DESK DRAWER OR TOOLBOX WHERE YOU CAN KEEP NAUGHTY THINGS, A BABYSITTER YOU TRUST, *Non-parent sleepwear,* A 'DO NOT DISTURB' SIGN TO HANG ON THE DOOR HANDLE, *a weather-strip lining the bottom of the bedroom door,* SEXY BED SHEETS THE KIDS AREN'T ALLOWED TO BE ON, AN 'OFF DUTY' RULE WHERE KIDS UNDERSTAND THAT THE ONLY ACCEPTABLE INTERRUPTION WOULD BE AN EMERGENCY

what if the kids catch you in the act?

WOMEN ARE OFTEN TOO DISTRACTED by their 'what if' fears to enjoy sex. Like 'What if my child walks in, gets scared and thinks, "DADDY'S KILLING MUMMY"?' For the record, fathers fear their sons walking in and thinking, 'DADDY'S BORING MUMMY!' Either way, it does happen. You thought the kids were asleep. You thought the door was locked. Now what?

If your kids are very young, the sights and sounds of sex probably will frighten them. Don't panic. Be matter-of-fact and tell them that mummy and daddy like to touch, hug and kiss each other differently when they're alone. Assure them that no one was hurt. Or bored.

If your kids are primary school age, they'll probably be more curious than scared. If you're comfortable, use this as a 'teachable moment'. Tell them children are created when love is expressed in a certain physical way. If you don't want to have a 'birds and the bees' conversation then cut to the chase and say, 'Everything's fine. We were having grown-up fun.' Either way, be brief, don't shame, and don't blame.

If your kids are pre-teens or teens, they know exactly what's going on. Now it's your turn to blush because I promise the only thing they'll feel stronger than embarrassment is revulsion. You have two options: stretch the truth so they don't have to hear anything they don't want ('We were just giving each other a massage') or just acknowledge the awkwardness of it all. Trust me, it'll be the shortest conversation you'll ever have. They'll make sure of that.

other sex busters

KIDS AREN'T THE ONLY THINGS that can kill your sex life. Sex can kill it, too. Ask a sex addict who cheats behind your back to get his fix. I'm not talking about affairs or one night stands. I'm talking about the millions of men and women (mostly men according to statistics) who put their relationships at risk because of their compulsive need for sex. The addictions include watching porn, cruising public parks/restrooms, trying to score in chat rooms, picking up sex workers or hustlers, having multiple affairs, voyeurism, solicitation, phone sex and masturbation.

ADDICTION OR PROBLEM

Personally, I think the word 'addiction' is used way too often to describe harmful habits. A problem isn't necessarily an addiction. Still, there are ways to tell. Sex addictions tend to have a progressive arc: a binge that creates the high, followed by guilt, regret and a promise to stop. Which is followed by an extraordinary hunger for the sexual activity, the creation of breathtakingly self-serving justifications for the destructive behaviour, and then the binge. Repeat, oh, five or six hundred times and you've got a full-fledged addiction.

When sex gets in the way of work, love or life it can grow from a problem to an addiction. When what you're doing starts doing you, when your want becomes a need, when the organizing principle of your life becomes getting a 'fix', you've got an addiction. And, might I add, a big one.

The essence of all addiction is the experience of powerlessness over a compulsive behaviour. Addicts get to a point where they want to stop, try and repeatedly fail. They suffer. They lose relationships, have difficulties with work, get arrested, have financial troubles, lose interest in non-sexual activities and end up with a rock-bottom self-esteem and an endless sense of despair.

When sex gets in the way of work, love or life it can grow from a problem to an addiction

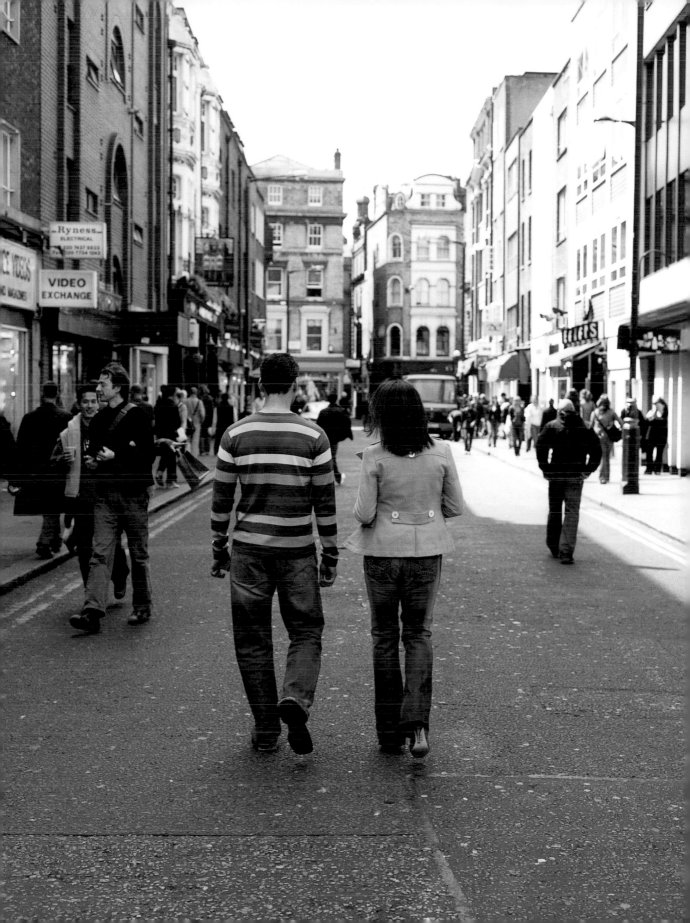

quiz: are you a sex addict?

Do you often feel powerless over your sexual behaviour?
Yes   (4)
No   (2)
Often   (3)

The worrisome behaviour has been going on for:
A few weeks   (2)
A few months   (3)
A few years   (4)

Have you lost friendships, relationships or jobs because of your sexual escapades?
No   (2)
I've come close   (3)
Yes   (4)

Have you ever been arrested or put yourself at risk of being arrested for your sexual activities?
No   (2)
Yes   (4)
I've come close   (3)

Have you ever left an important event (family reunion, work conference) to seek out sexual release?
Yes   (4)
No   (2)
Thought about it   (3)

Do you find yourself having to take more and more risks, needing more frequency and variety, to get the same kind of sexual/emotional high?
Yes   (4)
No   (2)
Sometimes   (3)

Are you keeping secrets about what you're doing or where you're going? Do you feel like you're leading a double life?
Yes   (4)
No   (2)
Starting to   (3)

Do you have a family history of substance abuse, pathological gambling, eating disorders or sexual compulsion?

Yes (4)
No (2)

Do you spend more than eleven hours a week in online sex chat rooms or downloading porn?

Yes (4)
No (2)

Have you masturbated so frequently and so hard that you've injured yourself?

Yes (4)
No (2)
Just the once (3)

Do you often masturbate at inappropriate times or places?

Yes (4)
No (2)
Sometimes (3)

Are you having a hard time paying bills because of the money you're spending on phone sex or porn?

Yes (4)
No (2)
Sometimes (3)

Does your sexual behaviour give you an incredible high followed by a lonely, despairing crash?

Yes (4)
No (2)
Sometimes (3)

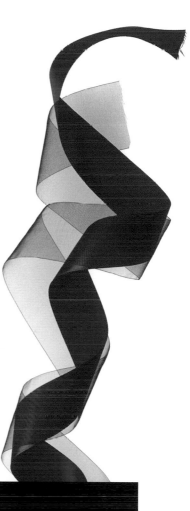

SCORE

0-26
You don't have a problem; you have a hobby.

27-39
If you're not worrying, START.

40-52
You might be a sex addict.

ASSESSMENT

IF YOUR RESULT IS OVER FORTY, HERE'S WHAT YOU NEED TO DO:

1.FIND A GOOD SEX THERAPIST: the British Association for Sexual and Relationship Therapy (www.basrt.org.uk) is a great place to start. They provide a 'Therapist Locator' by region. Or try www.relate.org.uk . They provide more sex therapy in the UK than any other organization.

2. ATTEND SEX ADDICTS ANONYMOUS MEETINGS. Their website (www.sexaa.org) lists meeting dates, times and locations throughout the UK

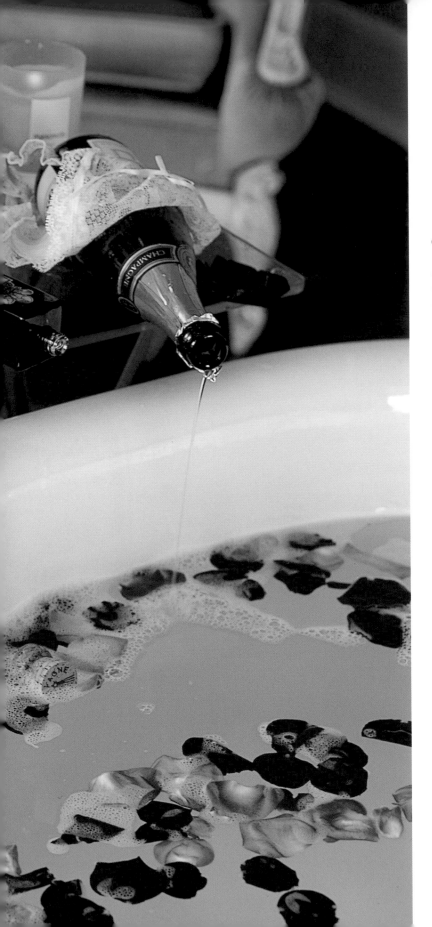

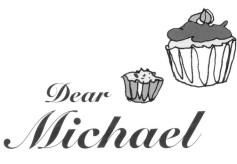

Dear *Michael*

MY BOYFRIEND AND I ARE IN A
COMMITTED RELATIONSHIP. WE HAVE A
GOOD SEX LIFE BUT IT ISN'T UNUSUAL
FOR ME TO WAKE UP AND FIND HIM
MASTURBATING. I'M HURT THAT HE'S
CHOOSING HIS HAND OVER ME. IT'S A
BIG TURN-OFF AND MAKES ME WANT
TO HAVE LESS AND LESS SEX. HOW CAN
I GET HIM TO STOP PLAYING WITH
HIMSELF AND PLAY MORE WITH ME?

Let me explain Manland: male hands
are going to migrate south whether
it's winter or summer, cold or hot,
single or not. And you know what?
Yours should, too. Sex is a way of
communicating. Don't look down on
self-expression. Anyway, your
boyfriend could be masturbating in
the morning for several reasons:

● He may not want to wake you.

● He may think you don't want to
have sex in the morning.

● He may have fantasies about you
that he doesn't feel comfortable
communicating. Masturbating gives
him the chance to play out the
fantasy.

 The next time he takes matters into his
own hands, I'd say the three words
every man lives to hear: 'Can I
watch?'

drink up or fall down

FOR SINGLE MEN AND WOMEN one of the biggest drawbacks to drinking too much is that it can make you think 'safe sex' is a padded headboard. For everyone else, the biggest negative is that you won't be able to perform. Winston Churchill proudly said he'd taken more out of alcohol than it had taken out of him. He clearly wasn't in the bedroom when he said it. Alcohol dulls the nerves that transmit sensations. It ups the desire but lowers the performance. In women it decreases normal lubrication and can lead to painful sex. In men, it can give you 'beer sex' or 'brewer's droop'. This means that the hardest thing you'll have to offer her is the bottle you're drinking out of.

Alcohol is not an aphrodisiac, but you'd be a fool not to recognize its power to melt away reservations, inhibitions and worries, the three pillars of awful sex. So yes, alcohol can be quite helpful in moderation. But what's moderation? Here's how to make sure the bottle doesn't throttle your sex life:

SIP, DON'T GULP. The liver metabolizes half an ounce of alcohol per hour (about the size of a regular drink). The faster you drink, the higher the blood alcohol concentration.

EAT WHEN YOU DRINK. Food can slow down the absorption rate by up to fifty per cent.

PHASE OUT THE FIZZ. Carbonated drinks speed up alcohol absorption so stay away from fizzy mixers.

HOSE IT DOWN. Drink a glass of water for every alcoholic drink you take. Alcohol dehydrates, which helps desensitize nerve endings. Water replenishes and flushes the toxins out.

Alcohol ups the desire but lowers the performance

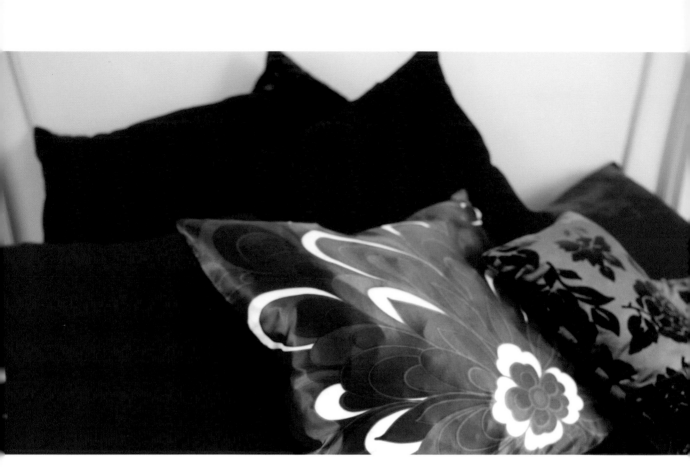

How much is too much?

Because the effects of alcohol vary by age, gender, weight, how much food you ate, and the medications you've taken, it's hard to estimate when one more drink will make sex a no-go. Still, since alcohol has the same effect in the sack that it has in the car, let's use the current UK Blood Alcohol Concentration limit for driving (80mg of alcohol per 100ml of blood). Sit down, guys. Bad news. After three pints of beer the only thing standing upright in your house will be the hoover. Ladies, it's worse for you. Your body contains less blood volume (because you generally weigh less), so drinking the same amount as a man will get you drunk faster.

other common sex busters
(and what to do about them)

THE BREATH OF DEATH

Sometimes it's the little things that can make your partner say 'NO' in five different languages. Like your breath. Many people consider kissing more intimate than intercourse. The delicacy of breathing somebody else's breath, the tenderness of tasting each other's essence – these are all sensitive, soul-sharing moments that can be ruined by one wrong whiff.

Unfortunately, you can't tell if you have bad breath on your own. Some people try cupping their hands to their nose to smell exhaled air. Others try licking and then smelling their wrist. None of these work. Your breath can smell like a sewer and you won't know it because the body becomes accustomed to its own odours. If your partner finally admits your breath is so bad her teeth duck every time you kiss her, here's what you need to do, besides brushing and flossing regularly:

● USE SPECIAL MOUTHWASHES. Avoid the ones with alcohol, which dry your mouth and make your breath even worse than it started out. Look for mouthwashes that contain chlorine dioxide, zinc ion, or sodium chlorite – they're the only formulas that neutralize the volatile sulphur compounds that cause bad breath. As you gargle, make an 'aaaaahh' sound. This will extend your tongue outwards, letting the mouthwash cover the back of the tongue where most of the bad breath-producing sulphur compounds do their dirty work.

● SCRAPE YOUR TONGUE. Use a tongue scraper daily. Try it after you've had chocolate or coffee. You won't believe what comes out.

● SUCK ON MINTS. They stimulate the flow of saliva and dilute bad breath-causing bacteria.

NOT TONIGHT, DEAR, I'VE GOT A HEADACHE

Some people get headaches after sex and/or orgasm, caused by the stress and spiking blood pressure. It's not very common, but usually nothing to worry about. Try taking a pain reliever before sex (but not aspirin because it promotes internal bleeding) and let sex build up more gradually. Studies show that 'quickies' are much more likely to give you a headache than 'gradual' sex because the blood pressure spike is so much more pronounced. If it happens regularly, see your doctor.

BREATHING HARD FOR ALL THE WRONG REASONS

Two thirds of the millions of people with asthma report unhappiness with their sex life. Check your bedding to make sure you don't have dust mites triggering the attacks. Use a bronchiodilator, which relaxes the muscles in the large and small airways, increasing ventilation. Also, change the time of day you have sex. Lungs function best in the late morning or early afternoon. The worst position for asthmatics? Having someone on top of you. Anything that increases pressure on the lungs can trigger an attack.

Foreplaying the future

Why don't women blink during foreplay? They don't have time. Slow him down by suggesting he gives you a massage. Here's what he should do: start at the head or feet, not the genitals. He should NOT give the kind of relaxing deep-muscle massage you'd get at a spa. You don't want to be relaxed; you want to be stimulated. He should focus on your skin, not your muscles. His hands should feel like feathers. Forget massage oils or lotions. He can stimulate the skin's nerves better with dry fingers.

HATE SEX WITH CONDOMS

There's nothing worse than a condom that's too big (ouch on the ego) or too small (ouch on the penis). Take the 'toilet tube' test to figure out if you need an extra-large condom. Your partner can help. Slide the tube of an empty roll of toilet paper over his erection. If it slides down to the base he doesn't need an extra large condom. If it gets stuck, it does! Remember, condom-makers rely much more on girth than length to determine their extra-large sizes.

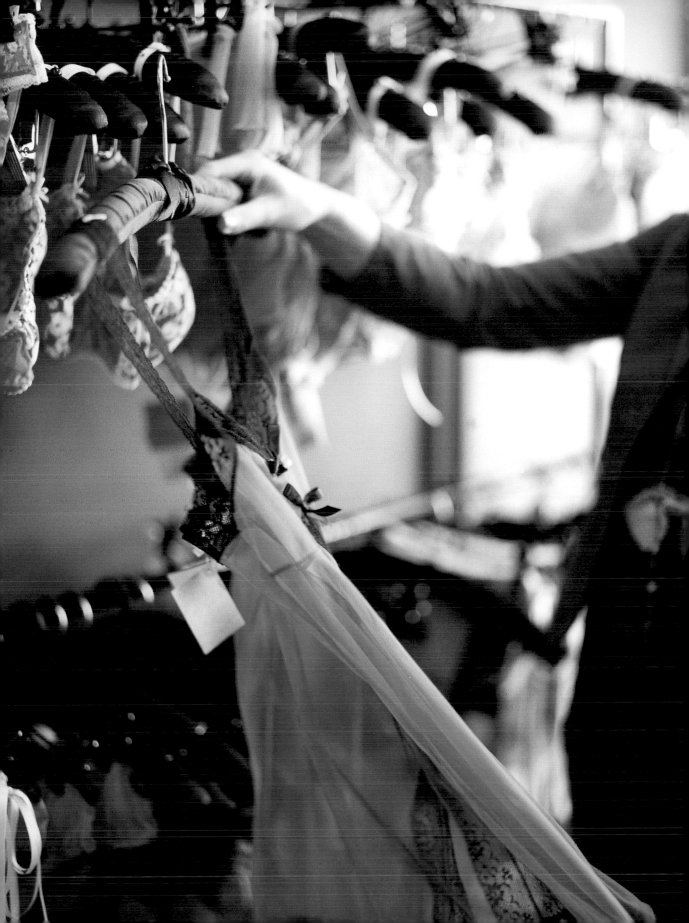

Heated emotions

Women want more emotional content while men want more physical excitement. There's a way to have both – by using sensual intimacy builders. You get her physically nude and she gets you emotionally naked. Everybody wins! Here are a few of the exercises we used on The Sex Inspectors. We call them 'emotional foreplay'. Interestingly, the men ended up liking it as much as the women.

● THE BELLY BUTTON BALANCE

Naked, lie side-by-side but in opposite directions (head to feet as opposed to head to head if you were sleeping). Put your right hand on each other's bellies, feeling your abdomens rise and fall as you breathe. After a while your breathing patterns will naturally coordinate, furthering the sense of oneness.

● LOVER'S STEEPLE

Sit across from each other, naked, with the tips of your fingers gently touching. Then stare into each other's eyes without saying a word. Staring into your partner's left eye seems to heighten the experience. In ancient times, sustained eye contact was considered a trespass into the other person's identity, so be careful – this is a powerful exercise.

● THE HEART HEATER

In bed, sit naked, facing each other, legs wrapped around each other's waist. Start by staring into each other's eyes in silence. Inhale in unison. Breathe at the same tempo, same time, same space. Breath and vision create union. Put your right hand on her heart. Put hers on yours. Feel each other's heartbeat. Close your eyes and feel the tenderness. Now look deeply into her left eye. Then into her right eye. Now change the breathing pattern. You exhale while she inhales. After a couple of minutes reverse. She inhales while you exhale. Syncing up the breath with the three points of contact (arms, legs, heart) deepens the sense of connection.

IT SMELLS DOWN THERE

Don't like going down on him because it smells funny? Buy him special underwear that whisks away sweat and body heat. Manufacturers have come up with a new fabric mixing cotton with an active ingredient called polyethylene vinyl alcohol. It keeps the skin one or two degrees cooler than regular cotton fabric, so you can ride him all over town enjoying that new man smell. Also, have him sprinkle talcum powder around his genitals before he goes to work. It will keep him dry and smelling fresh as a daisy.

IT'S DRY DOWN THERE

You want friction to heat things up, not burn them out. That's why using the right lubrication is so important. Lubes should help you make grand entrances and graceful exits without sacrificing a good grip. Here's what to look for:

● **TEXTURE AND SMOOTHNESS** Does it feel like saliva or cement? Is it hard to get off you? There are advantages to oil-based lubes but washing up afterwards isn't one of them. Stick to the water-soluble lubes, especially if you're using condoms (oil-based lubes will dissolve them). Silicone lube is expensive but feels exquisite.

● **TASTE AND SMELL** Does it smell like chemicals? Go for something neutral or something yummy.

● **DRYING FACTOR** Does it disappear quickly? There's nothing more annoying than constantly interrupting the fun to re-lubricate.

● **CONVENIENCE** Unless you want to stop the action to twist a cap open and then find a place to put the lid, I'd skip jars and go for bottles and tubes with easy-flip tops.

If you're allergic to lubes, avoid the ones that have skin-irritating ingredients like methyl, propyl paraben or Nonoxymol-9. Problem is, most lubes contain those ingredients, so you might want to try some of the new organic lubes. Rub it on the inside of the wrist, wait a day and see what happens.

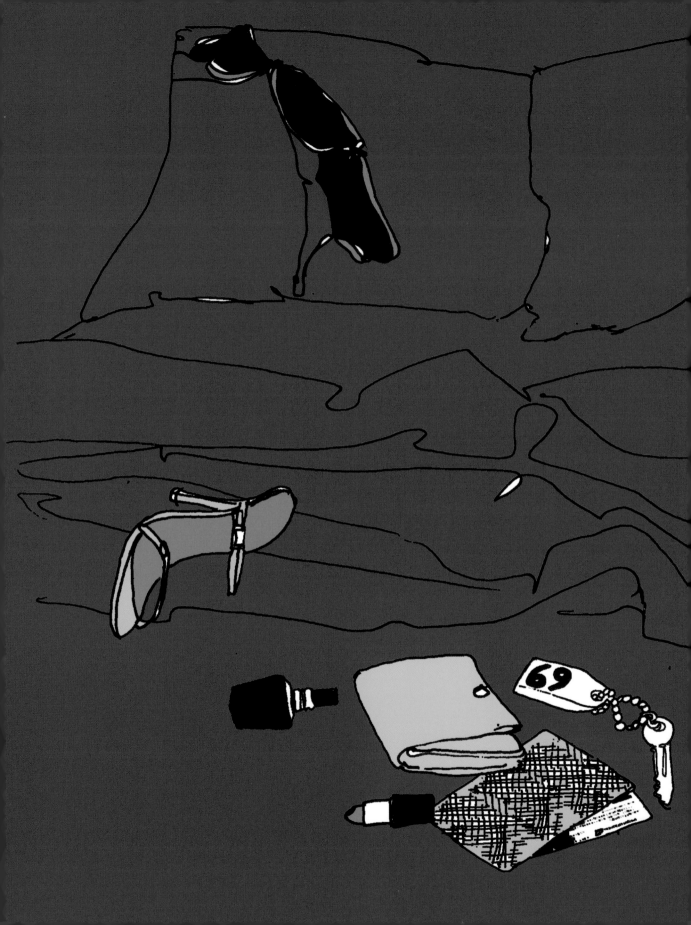

infidelity:
a survival
guide

Realistic solutions to resisting,
recovering and writing your
own relationship rules

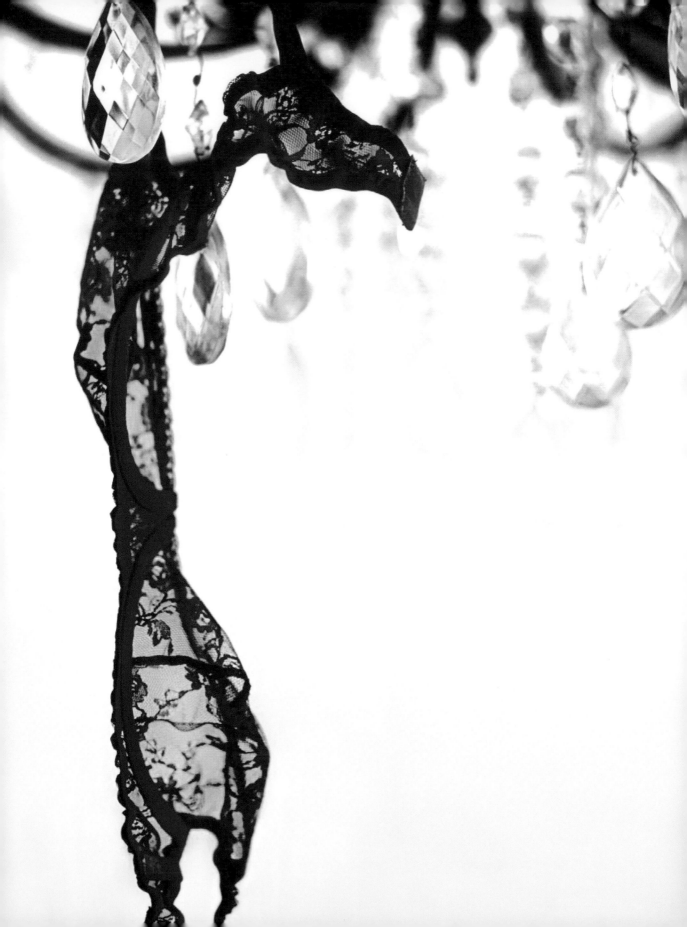

*O*F ALL THE CHAPTERS IN THIS BOOK, this one contains the least sex – ironic, since most people assume affairs are all about sex. Truth is, though, the majority aren't. A random one night stand (cue some clumsy fumbling and drunken moments of utter confusion when you 'come to' and suddenly wonder why the person whose lips and hips are pressed against yours bears no resemblance to your partner), might be just about sex. The opportunity was there, you fancied sex-without-strings and thought you wouldn't get caught, so took what was on offer. But long-term sex-only affairs – the sort which pop up in French films, where both get naked the second the door shuts, don't speak and finish each encounter by lighting a Gauloise and staring moodily out the window – are rare. The reason why they're rare is that despite puffing our chests out and boasting about being liberated and able to separate sex from love, blah blah blah, few people actually can.

In this chapter, I've tried to offer logical, non-judgemental advice on how to avoid, cope with and understand affairs. I've kept the focus mainly on the emotional ramifications because the rest of the book is packed with solutions to keep you both sexually satisfied.

his & hers affairs

WOMEN ARE WORSE AT IT THAN MEN, but not just because of all that Mars and Venus stuff. It appears our bodies produce a bonding hormone through vaginal stimulation which means the more we sleep with a guy, the more likely we are to want to play happy families. I hate generalizing about the sexes but women tend to have emotion-based affairs – usually as a result of feeling unhappy with their primary relationship – while men have sex-based affairs, even if they are happy at home. According to US therapist Shirley Glass, fifty-six per cent of men who have affairs say they are in happy relationships, but only thirty-four per cent of women say the same. Her affairs, therefore, are more threatening to the marriage because she is far more likely to be thinking about leaving to have an affair in the first place.

THE REAL REASON PEOPLE PLAY AROUND

Despite some gender differences, however, the real reason why people have affairs is this: to get something they're not getting from the relationship they're in. And since we're all individuals with our own quirky little needs, this means we have affairs for just about any reason at all. Some search for attention and admiration, others money and excitement. Some want to be told they're perfect, others want someone to let them show their faults. There's a lot more going on than the obvious bonus of being able to let loose sexually with someone who happens to share our penchant for a bit of bottom play. The incidence of affairs is rising. More of us are having them, on a more frequent basis. It's almost impossible to get survey statistics to match but an acceptable average is about forty-two per cent of us

The incidence of affairs is rising. More of us are having them, and on a more frequent basis

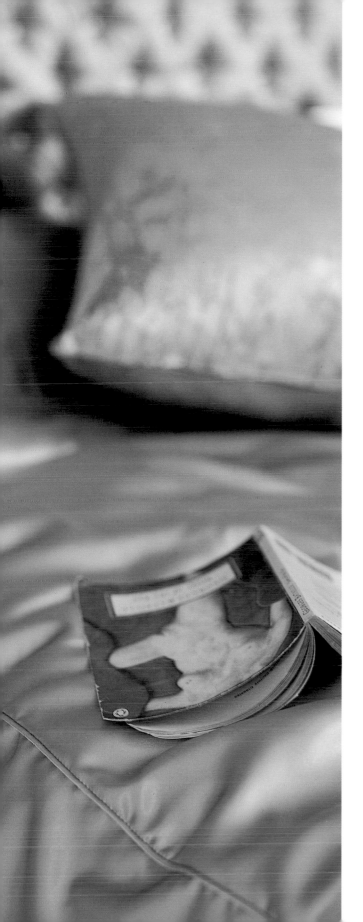

(male and female) cheat or have cheated. (Interestingly, another poll showed eighty-seven per cent of us are confident our partner is faithful and always has been. You do the maths …)

It's also never been easier to be unfaithful. Disappear to the loo with your phone and three minutes and one text message later, you've set up an illicit liaison. Our grandparents had to arrange secret assignations via the (nosey) secretary, snail-mail or through 'wrong number' phone calls, made and taken on the fixed phone in the hallway, within earshot of the person they were about to deceive. With today's technology you could organize twenty naughty nights in the time it took to organize a stolen brushing of lips.

ONE SIZE DOESN'T FIT ALL

If you're feeling distinctly nervous and/or oddly turned on by all this talk of being unfaithful, don't feel bad. Both reactions are entirely normal. Most of us abhor the thought of our partner having an affair but realize we might be susceptible to one, given certain circumstances.

As much as we might still try to squeeze ourselves into the

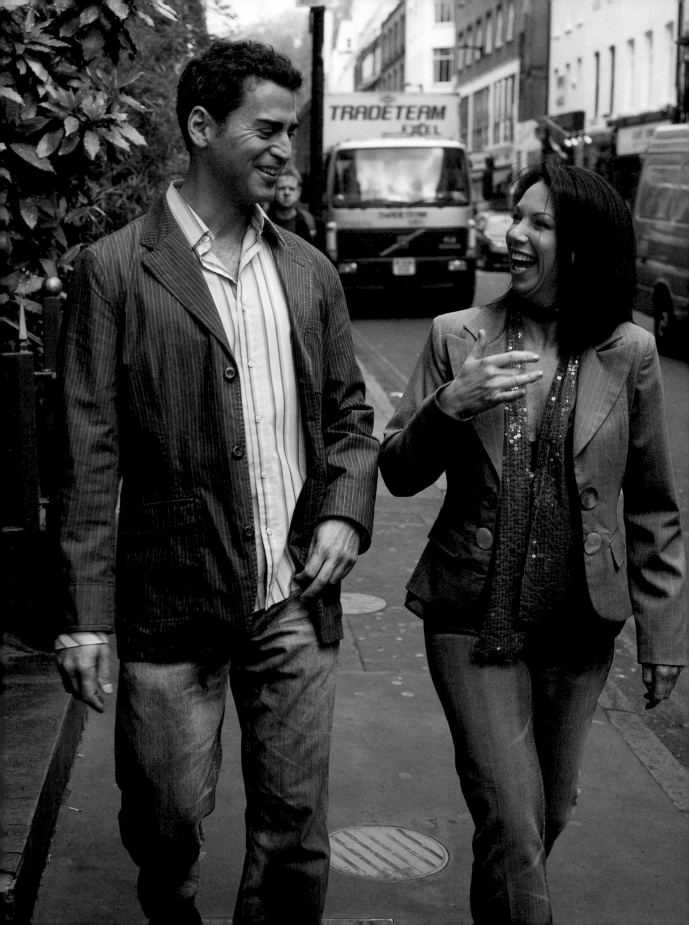

traditional model of monogamy, desperately pretending one-size-fits-all, anyone with more than one brain cell can see it's clearly not working for many people. The question is: what do we replace it with? Very few go down the dodgy 'open relationship' path because we're selfish (we want to be 'special' enough for our partner not to need other people to satisfy their needs) and idealistic (we want to find and be with someone who is so special, we won't fancy anyone else either). That's our hopeful, romantic side at work. A harder, cynical part of us recognizes even good long-term sex goes through boring patches and when that time comes, we'll also find it hard to resist when temptation inevitably presents itself.

WHY RISK EVERYTHING?

If you've got a pretty good idea that five-minute fumble could cost you your marriage, kids, friends and a lifestyle you love, why do it in the first place? One reason is we aren't able to think terribly clearly when in the grips of strong desire. Our body floods with persuasive hormones and all prompt us to do what nature intended: mate. The original idea behind all this was to populate the earth rather than get you in all sorts of trouble, but the feelings are just the same: primitive, powerful and pretty damn hard to ignore! There are apparent upsides to having an affair (see page 194) – why else would people do it? But there are many myths too (see page 192) which you should be aware of.

Question:
HOW DO I KNOW IF I'M HAVING AN AFFAIR?

Answer:
Ask yourself one simple question: if my partner saw me right now, would they be upset? Affairs aren't just about sex, they're about intimacy

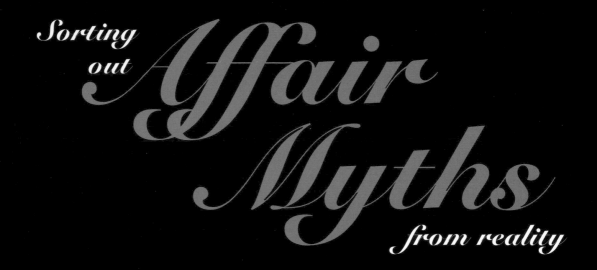

Sorting out Affair Myths from reality

'I was drunk and it just happened'

FALSE!

I've got lots of attached friends and we're all rather fond of a glass of wine (bottomless, that is). I've seen many of them sloshed, solo and surrounded by a plethora of available talent but – miraculously – it doesn't 'just happen' to them. Funny that. What people are really saying is the alcohol not only loosened their inhibitions, it caused them to make a poor judgement call. And since most of us have figured out, by age twelve, that's what alcohol does, wouldn't it have been logical to stop drinking once they felt themselves cross the line between merry and legless? Particularly if the hot little piece in the corner is inching closer on the bar stool. Come on. They didn't want to stop 'it' happening, and to carry on drinking armed them with a (weak) excuse.

AFFAIRS ARE SOMETIMES A GOOD WAY TO BRING A PROBLEM TO A HEAD

FALSE!
If you thought the problem was bad before the affair, try tackling it after one. An affair isn't the way to draw attention to a problem, talking is.

You should always confess

FALSE!

If you're confronted with solid evidence, yes. But if your partner has no idea and is unlikely to find out, it isn't always the best option. If you're owning up to relieve your guilt, don't – why drive a stake through your partner's heart to make yourself feel better? If you're truly sorry, stop the affair, perhaps see a therapist and become the sensitive, loving person your partner deserves.

MOST AFFAIRS DON'T LAST ONCE THEY'RE OUT IN THE OPEN

TRUE!

Secrecy and forbiddenness are the two main attractions – in other words, the appeal often isn't the person, it's the actual affair. There's also a high level of mistrust: you know they're capable of it, they did it with you! (And vice versa.) For an affair to survive, it has to be based primarily on love – which often isn't the case.

Few people leave their long-term partner to be with the affair person

TRUE!

Usually true but especially true if this isn't their first affair and they've been caught before. Why would they leave? They're getting security and stability from the person-at-home and erotically charged sex and excitement from you. And plenty more where you came from, honeybunch, if you're single and do see sense and make them choose. There are lots of other people with low self-esteem who are ready to settle for someone else's leftovers. (And yes, that is what you're doing.)

infidelity: a survival guide

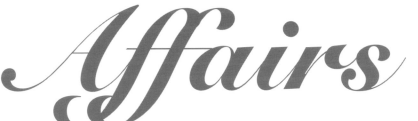

The reasons why people have Affairs

YOU CAN ASK THEM TO DO THINGS YOU WOULDN'T DREAM OF ASKING YOUR PARTNER. Your fantasy is to be chained to a dungeon wall and whipped into submission, your partner's idea of sexual nirvana is a candlelit dinner followed by sex in the missionary position. Under the duvet. If there are things you're desperate to do but know your partner won't be into, an affair with a kindred spirit seems like the solution. Some people don't necessarily even want their partners to satisfy all their cravings, secretly considering it 'beneath' her or him.

IT'S FORBIDDEN. Nothing like an 'open' relationship to ruin the 'thrill' of having an affair. Realizing this, some people assure their partners they won't mind if they play around, knowing full well that once given 'permission', the appeal dwindles. (Though still not one

I'd recommend – it could backfire spectacularly!) It's human nature to want what we can't have and there's nothing like doing something we shouldn't to trigger that 'Am I nervous or excited?' tummy wobble. The rush of hormones which accompanies risky behaviour can be more addictive than nicotine (and twice as dangerous).

YOUR PREVIOUSLY LAGGING LIBIDO IS SPECTACULARLY REVIVED. Nothing like fresh flesh to have everything standing to attention and even if you are astute enough to realize this too will fade, the instant gratification of boarding the rollercoaster at the starting gate can be irresistible.

YOU DON'T SEE EACH OTHER OFTEN. You're constantly left wanting more, which is in itself an aphrodisiac.

THERE'S A CONSTANT FEAR YOU MIGHT GET CAUGHT – YOU'RE RISKING EVERYTHING. For some people, the resulting guilt and nerves render them virtually incapable of performing sexually with their partner. Others find sex with their partner gets better because each guilty thrust reminds them they could lose the lot if they're not careful. Taking risks is exciting for lots of people.

Why affairs are never worth it

● Lots of people leave their partners after an affair, unable to cope with the consequences. You stand to lose a partner who loves you, the life you share, your children growing up, possibly your house and your possessions.

● The resulting resentment, anger and sadness often makes the relationship unworkable.

● You've broken the trust bond. That sense of 'you and I against the world' you once shared is gone.

● There is a loss of innocence. Partners will often sense something is wrong and the tension can be incredibly destructive.

● Affairs always involve lying and honesty is the basis of all good relationships.

If you're tempted, stop and picture your partner's face if/when they find out. Is it worth it?

emotional infidelity

THERE'S ALWAYS BEEN AN UNWRITTEN RULE that thou shalt not play tonsil-tennis with another person, allow them to put their hands or tongues on your parts or insert their bits into yours. The equation was simple: sex = infidelity. Now cheating has taken on a whole new meaning with emotional infidelity the new buzzword. But what, exactly, does it mean and, more importantly, is it putting your relationship at risk?

Emotional infidelity is all about being unfaithful to your partner without exchanging so much as a kiss. I'm talking that 'innocent' friendship with the guy at work/girl at the gym. You're just friends but you're much more than that in your fantasies. 'Intimacy' used to be something you shared with your husband or wife or long-term, live-in lover. Now we're sharing intimate parts of our lives with many of the opposite sex … and finding ourselves thinking, 'This guy/girl cares more about me than my partner does!' or 'He's quite nice. Perhaps he's a better option than what I've got?'

Emotional infidelity wasn't part of our parents' consciousness because women didn't work and most couples had a limited circle of friends. The only member of the opposite sex available to flirt with back then was either your best friend's husband or your husband's best friend. While plenty took up the option, most (rather sensibly) tried to resist. These days, not only is there more choice of people to have affairs with because we meet and mix with lots more people, but also the fuzzy line between 'affair' and 'harmless flirtation' is growing blurrier by the second.

We live in an extraordinary time. The rules applying to male/female friendships and male/female co-workers have never been so relaxed. But without rules there is usually chaos – particularly when you put men, women and alcohol into a room and remove their partners. (Which is your standard 'drink after work' or 'office party' type of scenario.) It's entirely usual for male and female friends to go to the

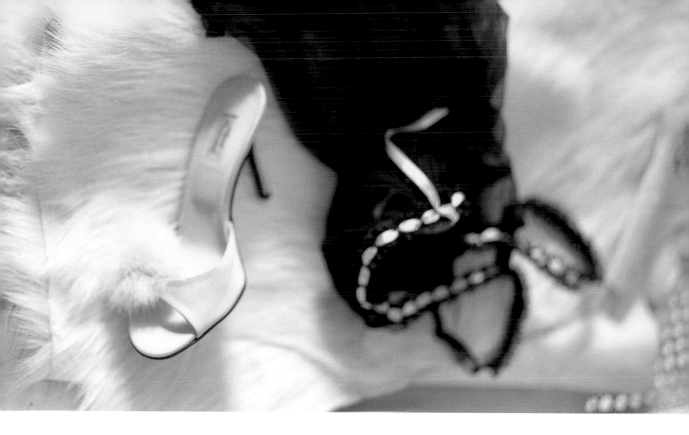

Emotional infidelity is all about being unfaithful to your partner without so much as exchanging a kiss

(temptingly dark) cinema; for opposite sex colleagues to travel for work conferences (staying in the same hotel, drinking together, eating together, growing closer and closer by the minute). All totally acceptable – except possibly to the poor old jealousy-ridden partner left behind. But they wouldn't dare question the situation, for fear of looking seriously uncool.

Add to this a myriad of new, deliciously secret ways to contact our new or old 'friends' – text, email, Friends Reunited (or is that Old Flames Reignited?) – and you can see why it's all got horribly out of control.

I'm not even for a nanosecond suggesting we ditch this new system and go back to the old one. The current freedom between the sexes is far healthier and it serves to keep both of you on your toes, given the constant competition. But there's embracing the new and taking advantage of it.

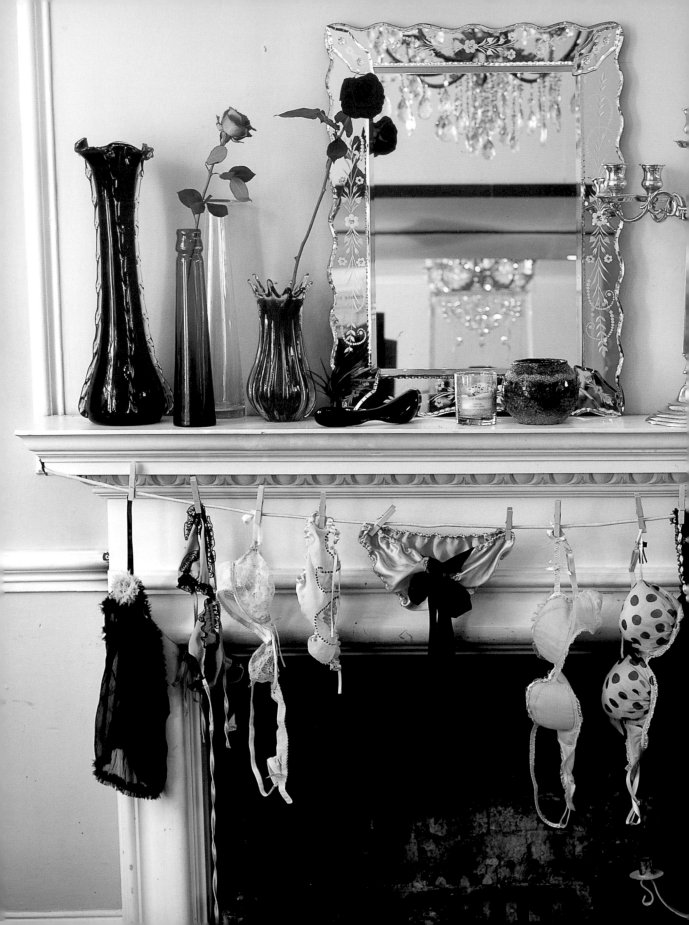

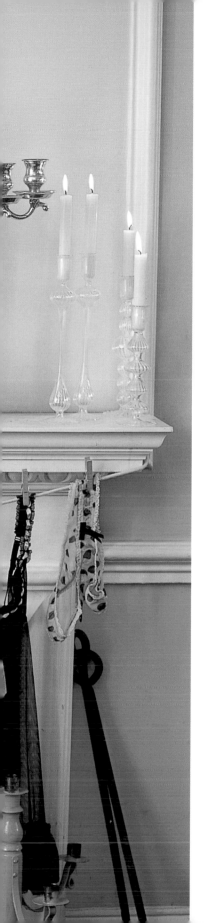

the new rules of fidelity

Want to be monogomous but not stifle each other?
This is what's worked for other couples.

1 WRITE YOUR OWN RULES

I don't have the answers for what your relationship could survive or what works for you, but I do think it's a very good idea to have a long, honest think about what's realistic behaviour to expect from each other. This will be based on your morals, personalities, expectations of fidelity, jealousy levels, type of relationship, religious beliefs, and much more. Some couples also take into account the level of temptation you're both exposed to. If your partner is a real head swiveller, works away from home on a regular basis and gets around twenty offers a day from supermodel types, your expectations might be different than those of a less than handsome lover who only meets one new person a year. Or it might make zero difference to you. I'm not suggesting for a minute that attractive partners with lots of temptation and opportunity should be excused from having flingettes. It's just that if we're truly honest (and at the risk of offending you, I'm trying to be), they probably are more likely to have an affair than someone who makes it to sixty without having received any offers at all.

It's an unromantic view, perhaps, but please don't think I'm in any way excusing or promoting infidelity. Nothing could be further from the truth. My father had an affair before marrying his second wife and I have been on both ends of it during my marriage and other relationships. There was a time I'd have wished my hands could leap out of the page, grabbing you by the throat for daring to think about being unfaithful. But being brittle, vigilant and unbending about infidelity didn't get me (or you) anywhere. Fact is, I've seen the nicest people in the world stray and not-so-nice people stay faithful yet cause more damage to their partners by being nasty on a daily basis.

2 DON'T CHECK PEOPLE OUT – PARTICULARLY FRIENDS – WHILE YOU'RE WITH YOUR PARTNER

I don't think there's anything wrong with sneaking a peek at the available eye candy when you're on your own. But seeing your much-loved partner exchange a 'wish we were single' look, is a tummy-turningly unpleasant experience. Their eyes slide up and down the person's body, their eyes meet and there's a definite moment of 'You're with her/him and I'm with him/her but if we were single, we'd be exchanging phone numbers in a heartbeat and saliva in the next.' It's a horrible moment realizing no matter how much our partner loves us, it doesn't stop them fancying other people. Or other people fancying them. If you both want to be trusted with attractive opposite sex friends, I'd avoid reminding each other of this vulnerability.

3 DON'T SHARE SECRETS YOU HAVEN'T ALREADY TOLD YOUR PARTNER

We're closest to the people who are closest to us. If you or your partner pick up the phone to talk to someone other than each other when something good or bad happens, you're in trouble. While it's perfectly acceptable to tell other close friends intimate details of your life, confiding stuff your partner doesn't know sends a very clear signal. It says to you and the person whose ear you're whispering into, 'I trust you/care about you/think you care about me, more than my partner.' If they or you have any ulterior motives, you're almost guaranteeing they'll be acted on.

DON'T DO ANYTHING WHICH INVOLVES LYING

Can you and do you tell your partner what you got up to with your friends? Is there anything you're glossing over or completely reinventing because you know they'd be upset to learn the truth? Once you start pre-planning and lying to create a time and place for that naughty flirt/meeting, you are an eyelash flutter away from taking it further.

5 DON'T HAVE REGULAR CONTACT WITH A PERSON YOUR PARTNER DOESN'T KNOW ABOUT

If you don't tell your partner about a flirtation or a friendship, it usually means you're going to act on it. Finding out your partner's been having lunch twice a week for two years with someone you've never heard of is shocking when it's a same sex friend. When it's an opposite sex friend, alarm bells clang so loudly, your late Aunt Mary, buried in Boston, does a turn. These lies of omission – the ones people try to get out of by saying, 'I didn't lie – you didn't ask me so I didn't tell you' – turn the innocent party into a paranoid, nervous wreck because they then feel they have to ask about every possible scenario or they won't find out what's really going on.

DON'T STEP OUTSIDE THE RULES YOU'VE MADE AS A COUPLE

Some couples might turn a blind eye to the odd stolen snog if there's no chance it'll embarrass the other person. Other couples know even a suspicion of it would result in them arriving home to find their possessions on the pavement. Most people are aware of what these rules are, spoken or unspoken. If you consider them acceptable and value your relationship, obey them.

7 DON'T HAVE ONE RULE FOR YOU, ONE RULE FOR THEM

It's not just because we want to have our cake and eat it too, it's because we know our own reasons and justifications: we don't have to convince ourselves it's innocent if it really is, so it seems okay. However, most of us are extremely good at deluding ourselves and pretending something's innocent when it's obvious a friendly pint and a packet of crisps isn't all we're after. No one's denying an illicit flirt is incredibly erotic, adding a much-needed zap to a boring work day or 'bored-now-but-don't-want-to-leave' relationship. But it's a bit like taking a sneaky puff on someone's cigarette when you've supposedly given up smoking: before you know it, you want a whole one to yourself then you're standing in the newsagents waiting to buy a packet. Loving with your heart but not your body can be extremely dangerous. Familiarity breeds lust, and if you feel yourself hovering on the brink and about to fall into an emotional abyss, take a step back from the friendship and have a good think about what could happen if you let it continue.

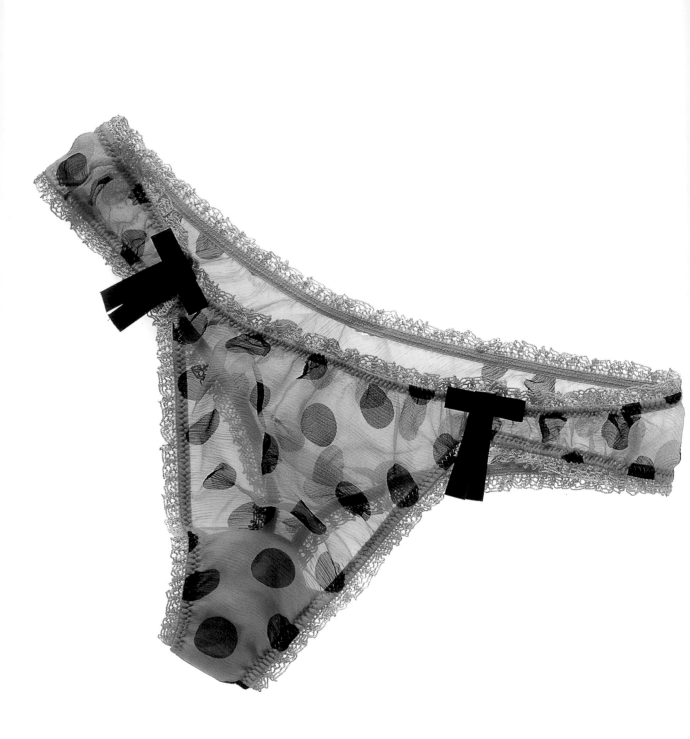

202
infidelity: a survival guide

Want a faithful partner?

I'm not suggesting you dump your partner if he scores a few points on this list, but research has thrown up a few areas of concern:

● THEY LIKE DRAMA. Some people are in raptures for weeks over an unexpected bunch of flowers, other people wouldn't bat an eyelid if offered a trip in a Lear jet. People who work in high drama professions (emergency medicine, banking, etc), or who need a big zap to keep stimulated, are more likely to stray.

● THEIR FRIENDS AND/OR WORKMATES PLAY AROUND. They're not exactly going to be the voice of reason and discourage them when tempted, are they now?

● THEIR FAMILY HAS A HISTORY OF AFFAIRS. Our parents' relationships are models on which we tend to build our own. If Mummy or Daddy played and strayed, we've learned that's what people do.

● THEIR JOB INVOLVES TRAVEL. I've always said when you've got the golden three – boredom, opportunity and sexual frustration – you're asking for trouble.

● THEY WORK CLOSELY WITH THE SAME TEAM. A big office might throw up more chances of them finding someone attractive but they don't get to know people as intimately as those working in a smaller group. The person your partner's most likely to run off with is a work colleague they see on a regular basis.

● THEY'RE RICH. Affairs cost money – all those hotel rooms to pay for, double the presents to buy, travel expenses, extra dinners out …

● THEY'RE POSH. The upper classes are notorious for having affairs because they tend to choose their spouse for different reasons than the rest of us. Breeding, money, status in society – all are often deemed more important long term than love. The real love interest is usually the bit on the side. (Sometimes they even marry them, like Charles and Camilla.)

● THEIR PERSONAL VALUE SYSTEM ALLOWS EXCEPTIONS. 'What goes on tour, stays on tour,' 'Exes don't count,' 'I was in another country,' 'I thought I loved them,' 'I thought you didn't love me anymore.' Some people figure it's okay to stray under certain circumstances.

should you give them another chance?

Crucial questions to ask yourself if your partner's had an affair and you couldn't cope with a repeat:

How seriously are they taking your vow to finish the relationship if it happens again?

Very often, saying, 'Honey I forgive you,' does nothing but set you up for another kick in the teeth later down the line. Why? By forgiving them, you're effectively giving them permission for a repeat performance. They got away with it once and the worst didn't happen, why wouldn't they get away with it again? Only if you make it abundantly clear that if you even get a sniff of anything suspicious, it's over – without any questions asked or answered – will they take you seriously. If you sense your partner's secretly thinking, 'Yeah, yeah,' when you're delivering this speech, forget it.

Have they done it before? Most people find out their

partner's been unfaithful after they've shagged half of Britain. If you're deadly serious about getting away with a bit on the side, it's easily done. It's only after they've been doing it continually and repetitively that they get cocky, slip up and you find out. Do some sleuthing. Ask questions. If this is true and they're into double figures, forget it.

What's happened to make them rethink their behaviour? Saying sorry won't guarantee faithfulness, ask for

hard evidence: what's made them change? People don't usually change unless something's happened to change them.

Are they genuinely sorry? Are they still contrite when

things are semi back to normal? They should be more upset by how much they've hurt you than you are hurt.

What state and stage was your relationship in when they cheated? If they were off with their personal trainer while you were still innocently floating on the New Love Cloud, it's unlikely they'll be able to resist when things become long-term and routine. If it happened during a particularly rocky patch – when even you were questioning if you'd last the distance – it's much easier to accept it and move on.

Can you understand the reason they did it, even if you can't forgive at this point? If the answer is yes, will the situation repeat itself? If it does, will you trust them to say no next time?

Do they deserve to be forgiven? How good is your relationship? If you've never been happier and this is the only black mark you could give it another chance (assuming they meet all the other criteria). But unless they're up there on the 'love of your life' list, why bother? Do you honestly both want the relationship to survive this?

Did you see the signs? If their confession is followed by you saying, 'I knew you weren't working late all those nights!' you've got a higher chance of surviving. If you saw the signs first time around, you're liable to notice if it happened again. If you didn't, how would you know if they're up to no good again? You've got no choice but to trust blindly (and look where that got you last time!).

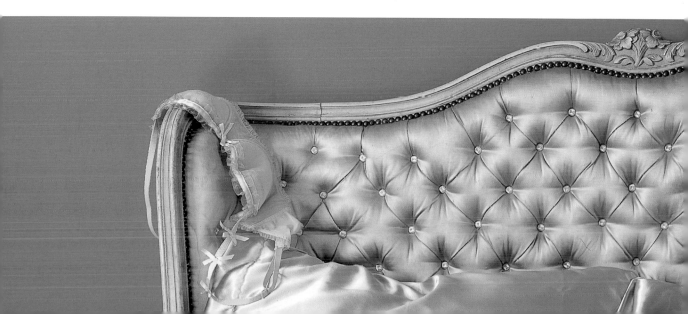

starting over again

Can you rescue what you had? After a serious affair, there's a loss of innocence and a scar, not to mention an influx of resentment, sadness and guilt. All make it impossible to recreate what you had before – but you can build a completely new relationship. Try this action plan:

● THE PERSON WHO HAD THE AFFAIR MOVES OUT If you don't want others to know, invent a plausible excuse. It's their problem where they go, but I'd suggest a very low budget hotel where they can think about what life would be like solo. If there are trust issues of what the person does while alone, book to see a counsellor to help you through. I'd strongly suggest this anyway. You need a separation for the seriousness of the situation to sink in.

● MEET IN A WEEK FOR AN HONEST DISCUSSION Both of you have had time without the other around to truly access your feelings. The person who had the affair needs to answer: 'What did I like about myself in the other relationship? What was missing that I was searching for?' The innocent person needs to see how their partner reacts to their pain. It's crippling at this stage. There's a permanent tape of what you think went on, playing over and over in your head. The person who had the affair should react sensitively to this pain and be willing to do anything to make it go away.

● ANSWER ANY QUESTIONS ASKED Refusing to talk about the affair or withholding details will be seen as protecting the person you had it with. This is such a no-no, it's often what causes people to say, 'You know what? I can't do this. It's over.' No matter how painful you think the answers might be, if you're asked a question, answer it. Do it honestly and tactfully but stick to the truth as much as possible. If they don't ask for details, though, don't offer any. Some people react well to knowing everything because they'd idealized the person and situation, and knowing they weren't perfect helps soothe them.

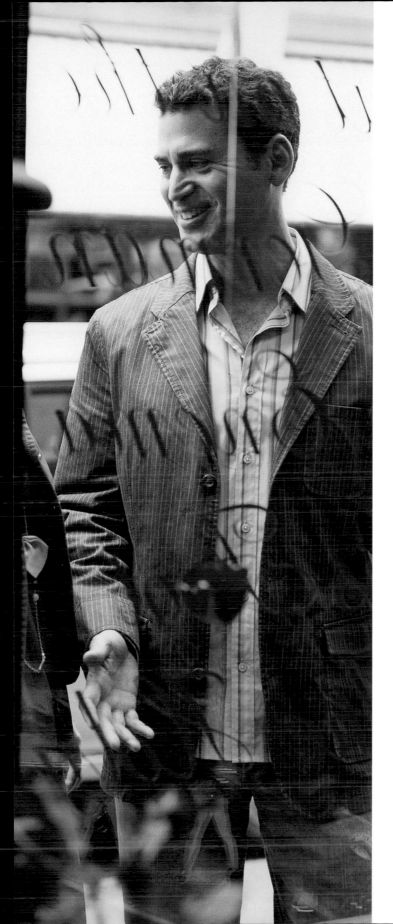

Others find knowing the literal ins-and-outs makes it too real – it really did happen, they haven't just imagined it. The wronged party gets to decide which way they'd like to handle it: the person who had the affair has no right to tell their partner what they think is best for them.

● **MOVE BACK IN BUT EXPECT A ROLLERCOASTER** The first two months will be hell but you should be back to some type of normality after then. Eventually – probably after about a year – you should be on a reasonably even keel. There will still be rough patches when the pain temporarily resurfaces but you've learnt how to handle it.

● **BE HONEST ABOUT EVERYTHING** If you had the affair and desperately regret it, this is the most crucial piece of advice I can give you: don't lie about even the smallest thing. Be scrupulous about reporting back. If you're going to be three minutes later than expected, phone. The shoes cost £300 not £50, the bus wasn't late, you popped into the pub for a quick one. You broke the trust bond – the only way to rebuild it is to be honest about everything.

affair-proof your relationship

As I said affairs are not just about sex – but it's certainly easier to resist temptation if you're having a grand old time at home. This is a fantastic way to do that:

A toybox for grown-ups

Parents are great at keeping kids amused, most providing enough toys, games and gadgets to keep the entire school entertained, let alone one bored five year old. As we get older, though, the toy box disappears. Somewhere along the line, a terribly sensible adult (probably God) decided people over the age of twenty-one should be more concerned with paying the mortgage and holding down a job than the pursuit of fun. After all, with all the joyous perks of adulthood (mind-numbing commutes, work pressure, the trials of parenting) what other possible stimulation could we need?

Well, for starters, how about something which is stress-free and enjoyable? In my opinion, the more pressured your life, the more toys you need to play with. We need more fun as grown-ups, not less! And never is this truer than in the bedroom. The longer you stay together, the bigger your sex toy box needs to be. Skip the bedside drawer – it's not big enough. Instead, invest in a stylish chest or basket which can sit at the base of the bed or slip under it. Start by stocking it with all the love-making basics: condoms, lubricant, blindfolds, scarves to tie each other up, books detailing position ideas, massage oil, glass-encased scented candles to put on the floor for flattering lighting, sexy CDs and DVDs, erotic lingerie, vibrators and other sex toys. Later on, add some fun lick-off body paint, erotic fiction to read to each other, a body massager which can be used on shoulders and feet as well as naughty bits, and maybe a fun set of fur-lined handcuffs. It's another way to keep you both focused on sex as something which is a treat, not a chore. It's too easy to start seeing it as yet another thing to tick off on the day's 'to do' list.

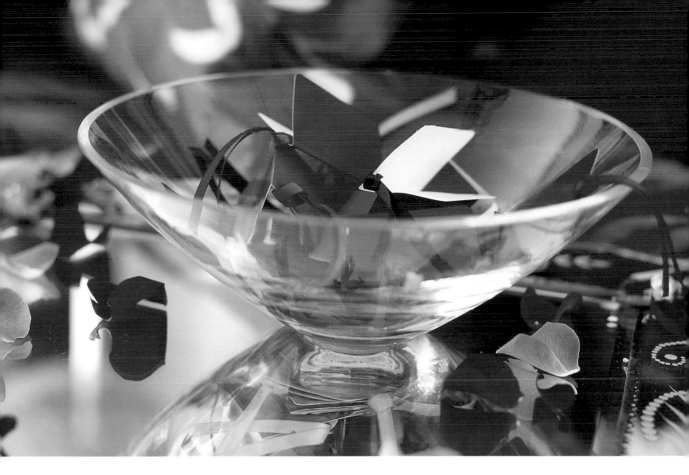

Lusty lucky dip

This works a treat because while it does involve the dreaded 'P' word (planning), once you've done the initial exercise, it's spontaneous sex from that point on. Ready? I want you both to write down ten new sexual things you'd like to try. You can do it there and then or take time to think about it. Aim for a mix of simple ideas, those which take more effort, the not-so-naughty ones, right through to wantonly wicked!

Once you've both completed your lists, swap and go through and approve or disapprove each other's suggestions. Try not to have a knee-jerk reaction. Like, is it really going to kill you to give it a whirl, just this once? Keep going until you've got ten agreed ideas each.

Fold up your suggestions and put them in a bowl. Once a week, one of you picks a suggestion out and does whatever it says. The joy is that both of you feel safe – you know it's something you're happy to try – but it's deliciously unpredictable as well. Take turns and you'll have twenty weeks of glorious treats!

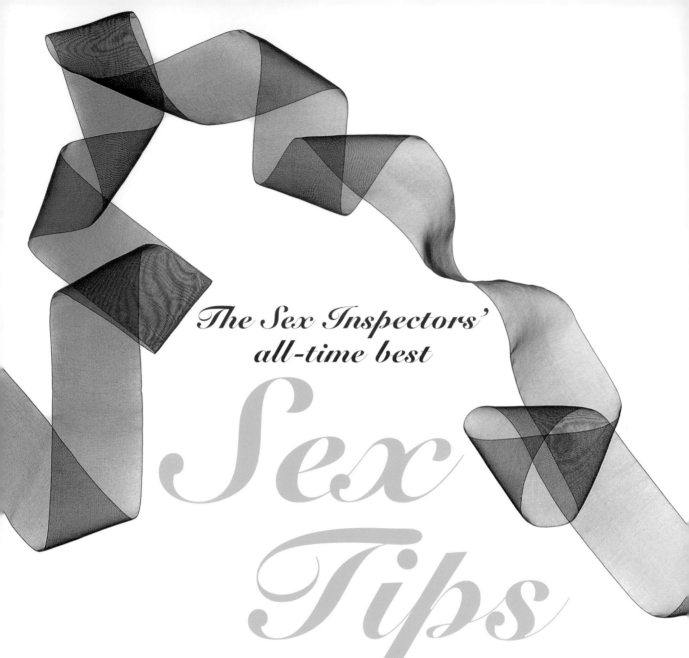

The Sex Inspectors'
all-time best

Sex
Tips

EASY, ACHIEVABLE
AND EFFECTIVE ADVICE
GUARANTEED TO LIVEN UP
YOUR RELATIONSHIP

Move around

Be active in bed. Don't lie there like a wilted plant waiting to be watered. Get on top, race to the bottom, fake right, go left and keep it moving. No matter what you're doing don't do it very long or very often. This will raise your energy levels and you'll leave your inhibitions behind.

TAKE A SEXUAL INVENTORY

Know what you've got in stock by taking your erotic temperature. Write down every fantasy, position, or act you can think of. To the right of each write 'cold, cool, lukewarm, warm, HOT'. Circle the temperature it brings out in you. Now, compare it to the ones your partner circled. Have a go at the things you've both circled as warm or hot and negotiate the rest.

Use your hands

Oral sex is no fun without wandering hands. Always get in a position where your hands are free to double the pleasure your mouth gives. You can, for example, put a left-hand finger in your partner's mouth while stroking their inner thighs with your right. Don't limit oral sex to your tongue and lips. Go out on limb!

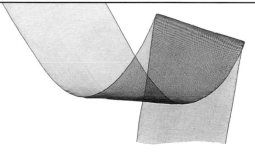

HEAT THINGS UP

If you want your sex life circling the globe get your blood circling your body. Heat promotes blood flow and so does exercise. So hit the gym, take a bath, and break out the hot water bottle.

GO FROM 'HO-HUM' TO 'OH, WOW!'

Pick a role, try a position, act out a fantasy. Sex will never be boring if you follow the Three E's: **Expand, Explore, Experiment.** Start with something as harmless as a blindfold. It'll give you a safe but exciting experience. 'Where did his hand go?' 'Where is her tongue heading?' You'll never know and that's the point. Creating anticipation is another way of making your partner feel new again. Free your mind; your bits will follow.

Try some emotional foreplay

Bridge the physicality and emotion of sex with Intimacy Builders. My favourite is The Heart Heater. Sit naked with legs wrapped around each other's waist. Stare into each other's eyes and breathe in unison. Put your right hand on each other's hearts and stay there for a few minutes. The three points of contact (legs, hands, heart) deepen a sense of unity and connection.

FOOD FIGHT!

Your pantry and fridge have more stuff to play with than an adult toy store (more textures, temperatures, flavours, shapes and sizes, too). You can't re-enact the scene from the movie *9 1/2 Weeks* all the time, but you can take bits and pieces of it. Drinking wine? In the middle of a deep kiss slowly squirt some of it from your mouth to your partner's. It's dead sexy. Cooking pasta? Each of you start nibbling from opposite ends, meet in the middle and seal it with a kiss. Be fun, be playful, be hungry!

Use some elbow grease

Sex without lubrication is like a salad without dressing. Yuck. Always keep high-quality lubes stashed in convenient places. And always use more than you think you need. Look for water-soluble, long lasting, neutral-smelling lubes in convenient flip-top bottles. Silicone lubes are expensive but they're also the best.

SQUEEZE YOURSELF INTO YOUR JEANS

The only proven way to exercise your way into mind-blowing sex is through Kegels – squeezing the pelvic floor muscles you use to stop urinating. They'll give men stronger erections and more lasting power. They'll give both sexes more powerful orgasms. So take your vagina to the gym and your penis to the health club, conveniently located in the car, your desk or wherever you're standing or sitting. Do 'The Squeeze & Hold' to a count of ten or 'The Butterfly' (flutter the muscles In half-second contractions).

STOP FOR A CHANGE OF PACE

The most effective method to help guys with premature ejaculation also happens to be the most enjoyable way for guys who just want to last longer and experience sex more fully. The best part is you graduate from self-masturbation to partner masturbation to intercourse in three easy steps: STOP when you're approaching the 'point of no return'. Let the urge to orgasm recede. Got it? Next step: As you approach 'the point of no return,' CHANGE your grip from the head to the shaft. You'll go from minuteman to 'As Long As I Want Man'.

HAVE A DIRTY WEEKEND AWAY EVERY SIX WEEKS

It doesn't have to be expensive, just take you somewhere the dishes, kids and bills aren't. If you can't manage a weekend, aim for one night, even camping in the back garden or a few stolen hours in a cheap hotel. A survey of US counsellors said time away together cures 90 per cent of couples who say they're in a rut. Schedule sex top of the list, not bottom. Instead of making it the last thing you do at night (with the enormous amounts of energy you have left – sure), make it what gets you springing out of bed, reenergised. Have chat-time and sex before you start dinner, switch the TV on and drift into zombie land. Have sex before you go out to that romantic dinner. Most people feel sleepy, not sexy, on a full stomach.

MAKE THE FIRST MOVE AS OFTEN AS POSSIBLE

If you always wait for your partner to instigate sex, you're missing out. Power is a huge turn-on and nothing feels sexier than being the one unzipping the trousers and promising the earth for having your wicked way. This can often zip-start the most sluggish libido, and your partner's pleasantly taken off guard.

Be great at oral

Oral sex is how the majority of people have their most intense orgasms. If you aren't sure your skills are top notch – and I mean unbearably torturously good -- polish up! And given that it's often the only way women orgasm with a partner, if a man refuses to give his partner oral sex it's worse than denying her chocolate on her birthday.

4 HIT THE BOOKS

You need three things for great long-term sex: knowledge (of how your body and your partner's body works), experience (practise makes perfect) and the right attitude (the ability to let go of inhibitions, not judge and not worry about what you look like). If you can throw in No 1 – a partner who is more appealing to you than a greasy bacon sandwich the day after the night before – you've got sex which will make you drunk with happiness.

5 *Choose the right partner*

By all means use your head and heart to make your choice for a life partner, but don't discount your groin. Love without lust is friendship and if you don't want to get naked when you first meet, imagine how you'll feel ten years on (yaaaaaaaawn). Chemistry is a crucial couple connection point: think of it as the skates which will help you glide through those rough patches.

6 TRY EVERYTHING (WITHIN REASON) ONCE

Your partner wants you to dress up as an Indian and sing 'Wigwambam' while simultaneously sucking their left toe? Well, we all beat to a different drum and if that's what does it for them, why not indulge them? So long as no one is being hurt physically or emotionally and it doesn't become a must-have fetish, anything goes. Don't judge. Judging guarantees your partner will never suggest doing anything vaguely interesting ever again.

SPEND TWICE AS MUCH TIME ON FOREPLAY AS YOU DO ON INTERCOURSE

Stop thinking of intercourse as 'sex' and foreplay as the stuff you do before you have intercourse. Intercourse needn't be the main course and your session doesn't have to end when it's over. Hands and tongues are far more dextrous than an erect penis and just as useful for producing pleasure. Get in the habit of having sessions without any intercourse by bringing each other to orgasm via oral sex or mutual masturbation.

Kiss more often

Because most people are orgasm focused, sex research tends to focus on this rather than things like kissing. Which could be a big mistake, according to US psychologist Geoffrey Miller. He's been studying why long-term couples kiss less as years go by and why people find kissing enjoyable in the first place. Bring back kissing, he says, and marriages will be rejuvenated and divorce rates reduced. I agree. Couples who ditch the hello's and goodbye's for 30-second 'proper' kisses tend to see extraordinary improvement, fast. That's one minute per day to improve your love life. Not that difficult, surely? Pay just as much attention to touch. Be emotionally generous outside the bedroom and you might find you have much more fun in it.

KEEP YOUR BRAIN STIMULATED

Famous sexologists Masters and Johnson discovered sexual pleasure involved the brain as much as the body in the 70s. They proclaimed sex 'psychophysiological' – which basically means if you get your attitude right, the impact on your body will be enormous. The brain is the biggest erogenous zone so you need to spend more time on 'brain sex' – fantasies, role-play, variety, surprise, anticipation – than you do massaging other, more obvious bits.

Don't finish where you started

While we'd love you to be treating each other to new sexual treats daily, real life often rudely intervenes to make things like work, children and household chores take priority over sex. (Shocking, we know.) When this happens, psychologically trick yourselves into thinking you've done something wild and outrageous by sticking to two rules. First up, don't finish where you start. This could mean you move to another room halfway through or if you start having sex in missionary in the bedroom, simply turn it around so you're facing the opposite end of the bed. Rule two: Do something you didn't do last time you had sex: a different position, clothes on instead of off, different music. Stick to these two rules and you've got a quick fix solution to keeping things good long term.

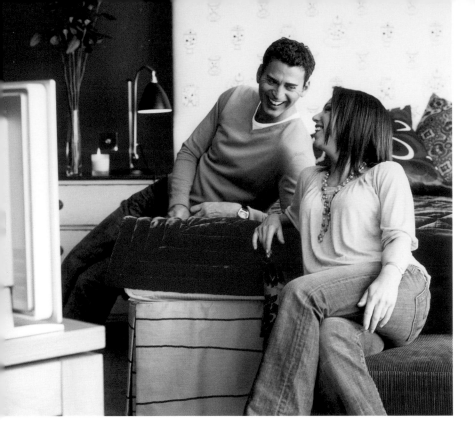
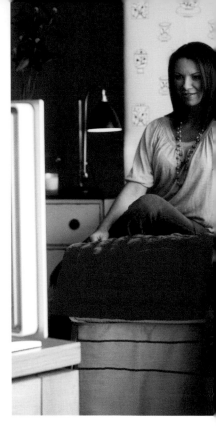

*I*F YOU DON'T PAY ATTENTION TO THE OPENING CREDITS of *The Sex Inspectors* you might miss something about me that's raised some eyebrows as well as some questions. What is it? Let's just say the only time I stare at a woman's chest is to read what's on her shirt.

So what can someone with my sexual orientation teach heterosexual couples about sex? It's a fair question. I think the answer lies in the special kinship between women and gay men. We share the same desires but not for the same men. We complement but never compete. My sexuality didn't just bring a unique point of view to the show but set up a natural trust and confidence that allowed me to do things a straight man would have had a harder time doing. Let's face it, when a man shows a woman sexual techniques it can look a little unsettling. My sexuality helped overcome that. Plus,

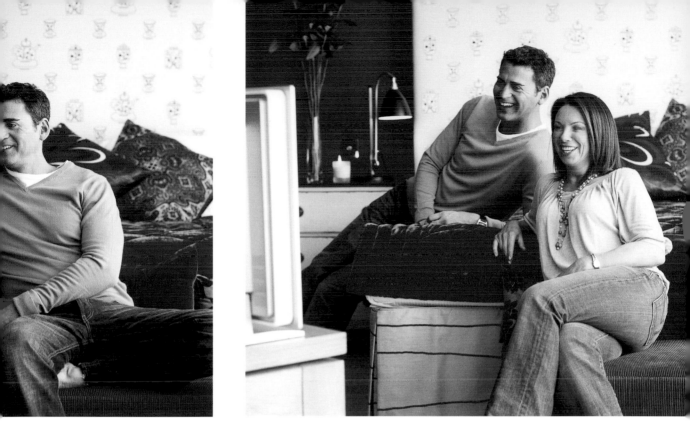

the guys never got jealous when I was alone with their women!

I have tremendous admiration for the couples that appeared on the show. Going on national television and admitting you have premature ejaculation is a pretty courageous thing to do. It takes a tough man to admit a weakness. And I'm proud that I'm part of a trailblazing show. Yes, there's plenty of sex on the television, but it often scandalizes, sanitizes or trivializes it. It never verbalizes it in a helpful way. *The Sex Inspectors* does just that. Our goal is to make people as comfortable talking about sex as they are about food. After all, how are you supposed to make a great dish if you can't talk about the ingredients!

We have witnessed desperate men, hopeless women and wrecked couples visibly bloom as they turned their sex lives around, often with just a few simple, practical tips. You can, too. Change is possible (and lots of fun). So watch the show, read this book, talk to your partner and put a little more spring in your mattress!

About the Authors

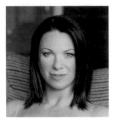

TRACEY COX is an international sex, body language and relationships expert. As well as *The Sex Inspectors*, her television credits include *Would Like to Meet*, *Under One Roof* and *Date Patrol*. Tracey's first book *Hot Sex* was an instant worldwide success and is now available in 140 countries. Tracey is also *Glamour* magazine's relationships coach, writes a weekly column for *Closer* and is resident sexpert for ivillage.com.

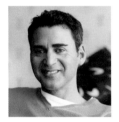

MICHAEL ALVEAR is the author of *Alexander The Fabulous: The Man Who Brought The World to Its Knees* and *Men Are Pigs But We Love Bacon*, a 'best of' collection of his nationally syndicated sex advice column, 'Need Wood? Tips for Getting Timber'. Michael is a frequent contributor to National Public Radio's 'All Things Considered' (America's version of Radio Four), and his culture critiques have appeared in *Newsweek*, *The New York Times*, *The Los Angeles Times* and many other national newspapers.

Supersex, Tracey Cox, Dorling Kindersley
Superflirt, Tracey Cox, Dorling Kindersley
Superdate, Tracey Cox, Dorling Kindersley
Hot Sex: How to Do It, Tracey Cox, Corgi
Hot Love, Tracey Cox, Corgi
Hot Relationships: How to Have One, Tracey Cox, Corgi
Men Are Pigs But We Love Bacon, Michael Alvear

resources

- *The Seven Principles for Making Marriage Work*, John Gottman, Orion
- *The New Male Sexuality*, Bernie Zilbergeld, Bantam
- *For Women Only: A Revolutionary Guide to Reclaiming Your Sex Life*, Jennifer and Laura Berman, Virago Press
- *The Sex-Starved Marriage*, Michele Weiner Davis, Simon & Schuster
- *The Sex Book*, Suzi Godson, Cassell
- *How to be a Great Lover*, Lou Paget, Piatkus Books
- *How to Give Her Absolute Pleasure: Totally Explicit Techniques Every Woman Wants Her Man to Know*, Lou Paget, Piatkus Books
- *The Big O: How to Have Them, Give Them, And Keep Them Coming*, Lou Paget, Piatkus Books
- *Hot Monogamy*, Patricia Love and Jo Robinson, Piatkus Books
- *O: The Intimate History of the Orgasm*, Jonathan Margolis, Arrow
- *The Fine Art of Erotic Talk: How to Entice, Excite and Enchant Your Lover With Words*, Bonnie Gabriel, Bantam USA
- *Coping with Premature Ejaculation: How to Overcome PE, Please Your Partner and Have Great Sex*, Michael E. Metz and Barry W. McCarthy, New Harbinger Publications
- *Passionate Marriage: Sex, Love and Intimacy in Emotionally Committed Relationships*, David Schnarch, Henry Holt
- *Ultimate Sex*, Anne Hooper, Dorling Kindersley
- *Erotic Home Videos: Create Your Own Adult Films*, Anna Span, Carlton Books

www.relate.org.uk
www.basrt.org.uk
www.traceycox.com

index

thanks ...

To Daisy Goodwin for asking us to present the show and by doing so, creating a lifelong friendship between us both.

To Julian Bellamy of Channel Four who had faith in all of us to produce a classy show on such an intimate topic.

To the team at Penguin and most particularly Kate Adams and Nikki Dupin, who have poured blood, sweat and tears into the project. To Natasha Law for stunning illustrations and likewise Chris Tubbs and Benoit Audureau for beautiful photography. To Alex Teal for interior styling, Sairey Stemp for styling and Jane Tyler for make-up. Thanks also to Becke Parker, Chantal Gibbs and Helen Reeve at Penguin Books and Cat Ledger at Talkback.

To everyone at Talkback Productions for producing such a ground-breaking television programme and especially to the two Steph's: Steph Harris for being such an inspired, supportive and talented Executive Producer and Steph Weatherill, our Series producer, who gave it her all (and managed to make it fun along the way).

To the rest of the team who also worked so hard: Production Executive Ian Liddington, Assistant Producers: Janet Chamberlain, Dominique Foster, Amy Sayer; Researchers: Gordon Maxwell, John Durbridge, Gemma Peakall; Directors: Claire Hobday, Rod Edge, Kate Morey, Ian Barnes, Helen Hill; Runners: Alex Robinson, Dan Holt; Production Manager Shaheen Gould; Production Coordinator Paula Sutherland; Production Secretary Jo Taylor; Crew: Camera Steve Court, Alistair McCormick; Sound Martin Leberl.

Michael: Applause also goes out to my sister Vicky Alvear Shecter for reminding me to keep my eye on the donut and not on the hole. And to Lisa McLeod for pointing out that there is, in fact, a donut to be looked at.

Tracey: Deepest thanks to my agent Vicki McIvor who continues to provide tireless and cheerful support and guidance throughout my life and to my family and friends who also give me so much pleasure.

Finally, we'd all like to thank the couples who so bravely opened up their lives to help the lives of others.

Penguin Books would like to thank Sam Roddick at Coco de Mer, Ed's Diner and The Soho Hotel.